T0309391

Evidence-Based
ACUPUNCTURE

ANNALS OF TRADITIONAL CHINESE MEDICINE

Series Editors: Ping-Chung Leung
(The Chinese University of Hong Kong, Hong Kong)
Charlie Changli Xue
(RMIT University, Australia)

Published

Volume 1   Chinese Medicine — Modern Practice
Edited by Ping-Chung Leung & Charlie Changli Xue
ISBN: 978-981-256-018-6
Publication date: February 2005   252 pp.

Volume 2   Current Review of Chinese Medicine: Quality Control of Herbs and
Herbal Material
Edited by Ping-Chung Leung, Harry Fong & Charlie Changli Xue
ISBN: 978-981-256-707-9
Publication date: May 2006   308 pp.

Volume 3   Alternative Treatment for Cancer
Edited by Ping-Chung Leung & Harry Fong
ISBN: 978-981-270-929-5
Publication date: November 2007   384 pp.

Volume 4   Healthy Aging
Edited by Ping-Chung Leung
ISBN: 978-981-4317-71-9
Publication date: October 2010   284 pp.

Forthcoming
Volume 6   Health, Wellbeing, Competence and Aging
Edited by Ping-Chung Leung
ISBN: 978-981-4425-66-7
Scheduled publication date: Spring 2013   Approx: 250 pp.

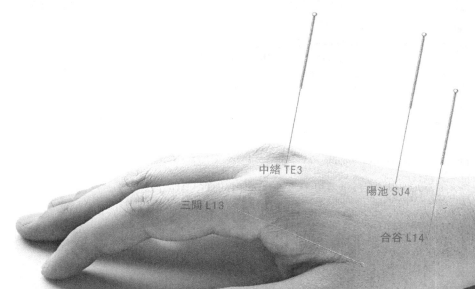

中緒 TE3

三間 L13

陽池 SJ4

合谷 L14

Evidence-Based
ACUPUNCTURE

Editor

Tang-Yi Liu
Shanghai University of Traditional Chinese Medicine, China

Ping-Chung Leung
The Chinese University of Hong Kong, Hong Kong

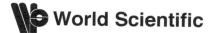 **World Scientific**

NEW JERSEY · LONDON · SINGAPORE · BEIJING · SHANGHAI · HONG KONG · TAIPEI · CHENNAI

Published by

World Scientific Publishing Co. Pte. Ltd.

5 Toh Tuck Link, Singapore 596224

USA office: 27 Warren Street, Suite 401-402, Hackensack, NJ 07601

UK office: 57 Shelton Street, Covent Garden, London WC2H 9HE

Library of Congress Cataloging-in-Publication Data
Liu, Tang-Yi.
  Evidence-based acupuncture / by Tang-Yi Liu, Ping-Chung Leung.
   p. ; cm. -- (Annals of traditional Chinese medicine ; v. 5)
  Includes bibliographical references and index.
  ISBN 978-9814324175 (hardcover : alk. paper)
  I. Leung, Ping-Chung, 1941– II. Title. III. Series: Annals of traditional
Chinese medicine ; v. 5.
  [DNLM: 1. Acupuncture Therapy--methods. 2. Evidence-Based Practice. WB 369]

  615.8'92--dc23

                                                          2012046517

British Library Cataloguing-in-Publication Data
A catalogue record for this book is available from the British Library.

Copyright © 2013 by World Scientific Publishing Co. Pte. Ltd.

All rights reserved. This book, or parts thereof, may not be reproduced in any form or by any means, electronic or mechanical, including photocopying, recording or any information storage and retrieval system now known or to be invented, without written permission from the Publisher.

For photocopying of material in this volume, please pay a copying fee through the Copyright Clearance Center, Inc., 222 Rosewood Drive, Danvers, MA 01923, USA. In this case permission to photocopy is not required from the publisher.

Typeset by Stallion Press
Email: enquiries@stallionpress.com

Printed in Singapore.

Editorial Board of the *Annals of Traditional Chinese Medicine*

Special Advisors:
Ke-Ji Chen (*China*)
Seung-Hoon Choi (*Philippines*)
David Eisenberg (*USA*)
Shi-Long Lai (*Hong Kong*)
Shichen Zhang (*Hong Kong*)
Xiaorui Zhang (*Switzerland*)

Chief Editors:
Ping-Chung Leung (*Hong Kong*)
Harry H.-S. Fong (*USA*)
Charlie Changli Xue (*Australia*)

Executive Editors:
William King-Fai Cheng (*Hong Kong*)
Sim-Kim Cheng (*Singapore*)
Chye-Tee Goh (*Singapore*)

Associate Editors:
Alan Bensoussan (*Australia*)
Paul Pui-Hay But (*Hong Kong*)
Bao-Cang Cai (*China*)
Kelvin K.-C. Chan (*Hong Kong*)
Timothy M. Chan (*USA*)
Pui-Kwong Chan (*USA*)
Wai-Yee Chan (*USA*)
Il-Moo Chang (*Korea*)
Yung-Hsien Chang (*Taiwan*)
Chun-Tao Che (*Hong Kong*)
Chieh-Fu Chen (*Taiwan*)
Yung-Chi Cheng (*USA*)
Moses Sing-Sum Chow (*Hong Kong*)
Kwok-Pui Fung (*Hong Kong*)

Ji-Sheng Han (*China*)
Joseph Tak-Fai Lau (*Hong Kong*)
Chun-Guang Li (*Australia*)
Liang Liu (*Hong Kong*)
David Story (*Australia*)
Frank Thien (*Australia*)
Ling-Ling Wang (*China*)
Kenji Watanabe (*Japan*)
Kin-Ping Wong (*USA*)
Peishan Xie (*China*)
Ping Xu (*China*)
Bing Zhang (*China*)
Zhong-Zhen Zhao (*Hong Kong*)

Contents

Preface to Series

Does Traditional Chinese Medicine Work?

History should be acknowledged and respected. Despite this, the historical value of Chinese medicine in China and some parts of Asia should not be used as the only important evidence of efficacy.

While clinical science has followed closely the principles of deductive research in science and developed its methodology of wide acceptance, there is a natural demand from both users and service providers that the same methodology be applied to the traditional art of healing. There should be only one scale for the measurement of efficacy. Thus, evidence-based medicine, which apparently is the only acceptable form of treatment, would also claim its sovereignty in Chinese medicine.

In spite of influential proponents and diligent practitioners, efforts relating to the application of evidence-based medicine methodology to Chinese medicine research have been slow and unimpressive. This should not come as a surprise. Evidence-based medicine requires the knowledge of the exact chemistry of the drug used, the exact physical or chemical activities involved and above all, the biological responses in the recipient. All these are not known. Working back from the black box of old historical records of efficacy requires huge resources and time, if at all possible. Insistence on this approach would result in either unending frustrations or utter desperation.

Parallel with the modern attempts, respectable Chinese medicine practitioners have unendingly and relentlessly cried out their objection to the evidence-based approach. They insisted that all the evidences were already there from the Classical Records. Forcing the classical applications through a rigid modern framework of scrutiny is artificially coating Chinese medicine with a scientific clothing that does not fit.

Thus, the modern proponents are facing an impasse when they rely totally on modern scientific concepts. The traditional converts are persisting to push their pilgrims of defense. Where do we stand so as to achieve the best results of harmonisation?

There must be a compromise somewhere. Classic evidences can be transformed into a universal language to be fairly evaluated and to be decided whether suitable for further research, using the deductive methodology or an innovative one after intelligent modifications.

There is a need for a platform on which a direction can be developed in the attempt to modernise the traditional art and science of healing, while remaining free and objective to utilise the decaying wisdom without prejudice.

With the growing demand for complementary/alternative medicine from the global public and a parallel interest from the service providers, there is an urgent need for the provision of valuable information in this area.

The Annals of Chinese Medicine is a timely serial publication responding to this need. It will be providing authoritative and current information about Chinese medicine in the areas of clinical trials, biological activities of herbs, education, research and quality control requirements. Contributors are invited to send in their reports and reviews to ensure quality and value. Clinicians and scientists who are willing to submit their valuable observations, resulting from their painstaking researches are welcome to send in their manuscripts. *The Annals of Chinese Medicine* has the objective of providing a lasting platform for all who concentrate their efforts on the modernization of Chinese medicine.

Professor Ping-Chung Leung
Institute of Chinese Medicine
The Chinese University of Hong Kong

Preface to Volume 5

After nearly 100 years of development, modern medicine has reached a significant maturity which covers comprehensive areas of education, health services, research and production. The practical side of modern medicine is always giving service or supporting production. Both education and research therefore are required to be conducted towards such supports, using methodologies acceptable to the users.

In the past 50 years, scientists have been using the reductionists' approach to explore new scientific methodologies and treatment options. For any form of treatment used against a pathological condition, the cause must be clearly known so as to allow a specifically targeted method of treatment to be planned, thence executed. For any form of disease treatment, scientists insist on the evidence-based practice. Many decades of clinical practice have established the evidence-based research methodology to be adopted as a golden rule, without which no treatment options could be recommended as a standard treatment.

The evidence-based clinical practice refers to a practice that has passed the tests of efficacy using a standard methodology. The essential criteria of the methodology include uniform intervention, carefully chosen patients selected for observation, meticulous follow-up of clinical changes after intervention, carefully chosen assessment parameters, objective analysis of resulting data and routine use of biostatistics to ensure a meaningful, reliable understanding, with which a valuable conclusion could be made for a more comprehensive utilization of the intervention. To date, without the evidence-based clinical practice screening, a treatment option could not be considered respectable. Without the evidence-based clinical practice screening, a traditional treatment practice could only be taken as an interesting traditional folklore.

Acupuncture has never passed the test. Acupuncture is widely practised and yet has not been considered Evidence-Based Practice.

In 1998, the National Institutes of Health in the United States (NIH) held a special conference with the aim of reaching a consensus about the use of acupuncture as a means to initiate analgesia. In this meeting, the consensus was established so that acupuncture is considered a practical method to deal with different forms of pain ever since.

It seems that the most respectable research institutions in the United States, NIH, have made exceptions in their professional assessment for scientific practice with reference to the area of acupuncture. What are the decisive factors that have affected NIH's attitude?

Proper explanations have never been made. I could make the following speculations. Firstly, we are all aware of the very long history of practice of using acupuncture as pain treatment. Excavations of ancient tombs have revealed metabolic and stone acupuncture pins and needles. The ancient practice unique for China would certainly gain respect. Secondly, with very few exceptions, acupuncture, as a very cheap practice, has demonstrated the highest level of safety. Thirdly, the practice is easy to learn and patients undergoing treatment do not experience much hardship and usually enjoy immediate results. Fourthly, with the rare exception of some special circumstantial background, acupuncture for pain treatment is usually given after other treatments fail or if the problem persists. Under such situations patients tend to be extra-receptive to the needles. For a traditional practice with good reputation, patients have little to demand for perfect explanations.

When one takes an objective analysis of acupuncture, one realizes that putting it to the standard evidence-based clinical trial with serious objectivity is something impossible. In order to make sure that the puncture site is the accurate one, the performer has to test the site and the depth of introduction, by gently manipulating the needle so that it initiates a special "sore" feeling. This maneuver precludes any attempt to "blind" the procedure, or to use "false" acupoints, or to use "placebo" needles. It is therefore impossible to insist on evidence-based clinical trails for acupuncture treatment before proceeding to recommend its use.

While application of the standard methodology to verify clinical efficacy is not possible, are there other ways of enriching the confidence of utilization?

In the past twenty years, new journals have appeared in China and clinicians are required to publish reports about their experience and observations. Our literature search to date reveal a lot of clinical records on the efficacy of acupuncture. A careful review of these reports in special areas would significantly serve the users. Moreover, laboratory studies of acupuncture using small animals are frequently done. Results would further contribute towards the understanding of the physiology involved.

The application of MRI studies during acupuncture has objectively proven that acupuncture initiates various neurotransmissions and that it acts through complicated neural pathways, and is not a myth or superstition. Han in China has done extensive research on the neurophysiology of acupuncture. He has made a most remarkable speculation about future research, making the observation that the physiology of acupuncture could be viewed as a complicated computer. Some of the basic connections and monitoring channels are known, while more are being explored. The functional changes related to neurological interactions are related to the basic connections. However, neurological interactions are affected by other humoral and immunological activates which are most complicated. The function of a computer depends on the establishment of a perfect balance after switching on the machine. Other functions of acupuncture (apart from neurological influences) could be equivalent to the unseen activities within the computer during the harmonizing period. These activities have definite material basis while the solid details would be difficult to reveal. Han's views could be an attitude to be adopted at this stage regarding the scientific understanding of acupuncture, where the internal harmony is probably maintained through multiple biological and molecular levels.

While acupuncture remains a pragmatic practice, and the number of practitioners is increasing, a book on the popular application of this treatment option would be welcome. Organization of this book is based on the following principles:

(1) A practical emphasis. That means the choice of topics is selected according to the popular use.
(2) The contents of each chapter would include literature review of past experience, related laboratory research, and personal opinions of the writer.

(3) A special emphasis would be given on the literature review, hoping that with such efforts, acupuncture practice could be more evidence-based.

(4) One of the writers would try to give objective and balanced views about the use of acupuncture to contribute towards clinical solutions. A balanced view is obviously necessary because acupuncture is not yet generally accepted as a standard treatment, while advocates tend to be over-energetic over acupuncture.

With such directions, this book will be welcome by the medical profession occupying the front line. Clinicians who expect acupuncture to serve them as a supplementary means of treatment, not only in the area of pain control, but also in other clinical areas of difficulty like allergy and immunological imbalance, will need this book. In addition, rehabilitation therapists will need this book to expand their knowledge and expand their armamentarium of treatment options.

Abbreviations

5-HIAA:	5-Hydroxyindole Acetic Acid
5-HT:	5-Hydroxytryptamine
6-OHDA:	6-Hydroxydopamine
a-ANAE:	Acid a-Naphthyl Acetate Esterase
ACA:	Anterior Cerebral Artery
Ach:	Acetylcholine
AChE:	Acetylcholinesterase
ACR:	American College of Rheumatology
ACTH:	Adrenocorticotropic Hormone
Ad:	Adrenaline
ALA:	Cerebral Anterior Lateral Association Area
ALS:	Anti-mouse Lymphocyte Serum
AP:	Action Potential
ARH:	Hypothalamic Arcuate Nucleus
ASO:	Antistrptolysin O
BCS:	Blood Cortisol
BOLD:	Blood Oxygen Level Dependent
BS:	Fasting Blood Glucose
cAMP:	Cyclic Adenosine Monophosphate
CB HRP:	Cholera Toxin B Subunit Conjugated Horseradish Peroxidase
C-CEP:	Cortical Evoked Potential
CCK:	Cholecystokinin
CFA:	Complete Freund's Adjuvant
CFS:	Chronic Fatigue Syndrome
cGMP:	Cyclic Guanosine μonophosphate
CHD:	Coronary Heart Disease

CIC: Circulating Immune Complex
CL: Central lateral
CM: Cerebral Motor
CNS: Central Nervous System
COR: Cortisol
CRP: C-Reactive Protein
CRH: Corticotropin-Releasing Hormone
CT: Computed Tomography
CV: Conception Vessel
DA: Dopamine
DAS 28:   Disease Activity Score using the 28 joint counts
DRN: Dorsal Raphe Nucleus
E2:   Estradiol
E3:   Estriol
EA: Electro-Acupuncture
EAA: Electro-Acupuncture Analgesia
EMG: Electromyography
ESR: erythrocyte sedimentation rate
FDG: [18F]2-Fluoro-2-deoxy-D-glucose
FEV1.0:   Forced Expiratory Volume in 1.0 s
FG: Fibrinogen
fMRI: Functional Magnetic Resonance Imaging
FSH: Follicle Stimulating Hormone
FUS: Female Urethral Syndrome
FVC: Forced Vital Capacity
GABA: g-Aminobutyric Acid
GH: Growth Hormone
GHRH: Growth Hormone Releasing Hormone
GnRH: Gonadotropin-Releasing Hormone
GP: Globlus Pallidus
GSN: Greater Splanchnic Nerve
GV: Governor Vessel
HPA: Hypothalamic — Pituitary — Adrenal
HPOA: Hypothalamic — Pituitary — Ovarian Axis
HRPAS: Heart Rate Power Spectral Analysis
HRV: Heart Rate Variability

HVA:	Homovanillic Acid
IFN- :	Interferon-Gamma
IL-4:	Interleukin-4
INS:	Insulin
LPO:	lipid peroxidase
I-PSS:	International Prostate Symptom Score
Ir-SP:	Immunoreactive Substance P
LAK:	Lymphokine Activated Killer
LH:	Luteinizing Hormone
LSZ:	Lysozyme
MCA:	Middle Cerebral Artery
MCAO:	Middle Cerebral Artery Occlusion,
MEP:	Motor Evoked Potential
MFB:	Medial Forebrain Bundle
MHC:	Major Histocompatibility Complex
NA:	Noradrenaline
NE:	Norepinephrine
NIH:	National Institutes of Health
NK cells:	Natural Killer Cells
NKT:	Natural Killer T Cells
NRM:	Nucleus Raphe Magnus
NS:	Nociceptive Specific
OFQ:	Nociceptin/Orphanin FQ
P:	Progesterone
PAG:	Periaquaductal Gray
PBN:	Bridge Periventricular Nucleus
PCA:	Posterior Cerebral Artery
pCPA:	p-Chlorophenylalanine
PEFR:	Peak Expiratory Flow Rate
PET:	Positron Emission Tomography
PET:	Positron Emission Tomography
Pf:	Parafascicular
PI:	pulsatility index
PRL:	Prolactin
PWM:	Pokeweed Mitogen
RA:	Rheumatoid Arthritis

RBC-C3bRR: C3b Receptor Rosette
RBC-ICR: Immune Complex Rosette Rate of Red Blood Cells
RF: Rheumatoid Factor
RI: resistive index
RN: Red Nucleus
RVM: Rostral-Ventro-Medial
SA: Sensorimotor Area
S-Am: Salivary Amylase
SCS: Salivary Cortisol
SEP: Somatosensory Evoked Potentials
SG: Substantia Gelatinosa
SI: Primary Somatosensory Area
SII: Secondary Somatosensory Area II
SM: Sensorimotor
SOD: Superoxide Dismutase
SPECT: Single Photon Emission Computer Tomography
T: Testosterone
TC: Total Cholesterol
TCA: Traditional Chinese Acupuncture
TCD: Transcranial Doppler
TCM: Chinese Traditional Medicine
TG: Triglyceride
Th1:   T Helper
TRH: Thyrotropin-Releasing Hormone
TSH: Thyroid Stimulating Hormone
Tyr: Tyrosine
UC: Ulcerative Colitis
US: Urethral Syndrome
VLO: Ventrolateral Orbital
VPAG: Ventral Periaqueductal Gray
WDR: Wide-Dynamic-Record
WHO: World Health Organization

Section I
Physiological Basis

Chapter 1

Acupuncture for Pain Control

Abstract

The most important clinical application of acupuncture is for the control of pain, particularly when the pain arises from musculoskeletal pathologies or conditions related to the head and neck regions. Acupuncture experts have accumulated vast experiences on the treatment of pain of different nature and affecting different regions of the body. Before discussing the practical aspects of acupuncture for pain control, it is important to understand the physiological basis of the pain control mechanisms. Neurophysiology is still a developing field, and the complexity of the neuro-anatomy and complicated functional pathways of sensory conduction and interpretation have limited the depth of the knowledge needed for the explanation of acupuncture analgesia. This chapter provides the information already established concerning the different parts of the central and peripheral nervous systems involved in pain perceptions and control, the neurotransmitters involved, the regulatory pathways, physiological theories and influences of electrical stimulation.

Keywords: Pain Control; Acupuncture Analgesia; Anesthesia.

1.1 The Central Nervous System

1.1.1 *The cerebral cortex*

It has been shown in many experiments that the cerebral cortex takes part in the pain control process of acupuncture. At present, research on the mechanism of cerebral cortex in pain control by acupuncture are concentrated on the following areas:

Acupuncture analgesia occurring directly at the cerebral cortex level

Experimental evidence include:
(1) Observing the behavioral changes in rat before and after removal of the cortex, and using nociceptive stimulation according to the operational conditioned response method, it could be demonstrated that the cerebral cortex takes part in the mechanism of pain control in acupuncture (Xu *et al.*, 1980).
(2) Taking 45 cats and basing on the background of spontaneous discharges of 244 body sensory neurons, observations were conducted to see the effect of nociceptive stimulations and hair touching stimulation on sensory neuron discharges and the influence of electrical acupuncture. Results showed that of the 244 sensory neurons, 50 responded to nociceptive stimulation (20.5%); 36 showed up-word discharges (14.8%), while 14 showed down-word discharges (5.7%); 11 cases of up-word discharges showed only restrained effect, which led to a decrease of emission rate (81.9%) (Xu *et al.*, 1984).
(3) Electrolytic damage to the Sm II area of the cerebral cortex could weaken the effect of acupuncture (Liu *et al.*, 1996).

Descending regulating mechanism from the cerebral cortex was found in acupuncture process

Experimental evidence included:

Using a cat as an experimental target, and by applying glass microelectrode for extracellular recording of neuron discharge from the intralaminar nucleus group (Parafascicular (Pf), Cerebral Motor (CM) and Central lateral (CL)) in the medullary lamina, and using electrical pulse to stimulate superficial fibular nerve as a means of nociceptive stimulant, the following were observed:
(1) After applying acupuncture, the nociceptive responses of most neurons of Pf, CM and CL were weakened by various degrees.

(2) After using g-aminobutyric acid (GABA) partially to delay S II area, the nociceptive response of most neurons of Pf or CL were not restrained by acupuncture. This indicates that the analgesia effect of acupuncture was related to the intact S II area, suggesting that under physiological state, the involvement of S II area's descending activity produced and maintained the acupuncture analgesia of the neurons of the three groups of nuclei in the thalamus.

(3) Employing the method of antidromic action potential, it was shown that in S II area there were projecting neurons directly facing towards CM and acupuncture could activate these neurons and restrain their nociceptive response, elevating their excitement and restraining the afferent of nociceptive message (Xu *et al.*, 1989).

(4) Using glass microelectrode extracellular recording method, it was observed that acupuncturing ST36 and GB30, could activate S II neurons (Xu *et al.*, 1984).

(5) There were other experiments that show that Sm II regulated and controlled Nucleus Raphe Magnus (NRM) by means of nucleus accumbens and habenular body, which are closely related to marginal mesencephalic system, and analgesia was achieved at the spinal cord level through the descending action of dorsolateral fasciculus of spinal cord (Liu, 1996).

Relationship between acupuncture analgesia and acupoint projections in the cerebral cortex

Using a strong electrical pulse to stimulate a cat's visceral nerve led to the excitement of A δ fibers and C type fibers. It was possible to record multiphase evoked potential (mainly scattered around anterior-middle part of the post sigmoid gyrus, i.e. the projection area of the greater splanchnic nerves). Applying acupuncture on "PC 6" (*Neiguan*) or the median nerve could induce electric potential of the cerebral cortex of which the major response amplitude of maximum evoked potential concentrates on the rear middle part of the post sigmoid gyrus, suggesting that this is an area where the sensory projection area of "PC 6" lies. Thus the sensory projection areas of acupoint PC 6 and greater splanchnic nerves are widely scattered on the post sigmoid gyrus, a criss-cross existence where many units stimulate greater splanchnic nerves and "PC 6" acupoint would all produce responses. When acupuncture was used to stimulate the projection area of cortical "PC 6", it would restrain evoked potential discharges of the cortical greater splanchnic nerve area, indicating that the restrain possibly worked through the projection area of cortical "PC 6" (Chen *et al.*,1980; Zhang *et al.*, 1980a).

Possible mechanism leading to incomplete pain control
with acupuncture

The stimulation of somatosensory area I (Sm I) of the cerebral cortex could be made through the head of caudate nucleus of extrapyramidal tract system to achieve certain regulating and control effect, strengthening acupuncture analgesia. It could also work through the pyramidal tract at the spinal cord level, directly restraining the input of nociceptive messages, leading to analgesia. The pyramidal tract and extrapyramidal tract system have opposite effects on acupuncture analgesia, whereby the function of any one of them could make a change in the effects of acupuncture analgesia. This may be one of the mechanisms that cause the incomplete acupuncture analgesia (Liu, 1996).

1.2 The Function of Cerebral Limbic System
in Acupuncture Analgesia

Acupuncture stimulation on domestic rabbit showed that the caudate nucleus, septal area, hippocampus, amygdaloidal nucleus, lateral preoptic area and mesencephalon aqueduct surrounding periaquaductal gray (PAG) of the limbic structure have important functions in acupuncture analgesia. By injecting micro-quantities of opiate receptor antagonist Naloxone to the caudate nucleus, septal area, hippocampus, preoptic area or PAG, the effect of acupuncture would be partial blockage. The achievement of acupuncture analgesia is made via high affinity binding site of opiate receptor subtype. In the course of acupuncture analgesia, the release of opioid peptide was increased in the caudate nucleus, septal area, preoptic area and PAG. It was proved that the opioid peptide system of the above mentioned brain areas, from presynaptic level to receptor level, all take part in acupuncture analgesia (Cao, 1989).

1.3 Function of Diencephalon in Acupuncture Analgesia

1.3.1 *Thalamus*

(1) In the experiment to observe the central inferior nucleus of the thalamus, microdoses of Lidocaine, a local anesthetic, was injected to find out the analgesia effect under different intensities of acupuncture. It was found that injecting local anesthetic into the central inferior nucleus obviously weakened the inhibition effect of acupuncture but it did not affect the restrained effect of weak acupuncture. No effects were found by injecting local anesthetic to other structures adjacent to central inferior nucleus of the thalamus. This result suggested that the central inferior nucleus of the thalamus played an important role in the central mechanism of analgesia (Wang *et al.*, 2006).

(2) Other experiments to explore the function of palladium in acupuncture analgesia using behavioral science and electrophysiological methods were reported. The results indicated that acupuncture could raise a large mouse's leg retraction threshold, inhibiting the nociceptive response of thalamus Pf neurons. When the Globlus Pallidus (GP) was damaged, acupuncture analgesia was weakened partially, without being completely blocked (Wu *et al.*, 2002).

(3) Using the glass microelectrode extracellular recording method, it was observed that the Sm neurons of a mouse responded to hand needling stimulation; the longer the serial length and the more repetitions of the stimulation, the stronger the responses. These results suggested that acupuncture and the nociceptive mechanical stimulation have the same kind of attributes. In conclusion, Sm might have important function in the production of analgesia following the detection of needling feeling and the excitement of small fibers by acupuncture (Yang *et al.*, 2001).

1.3.2 *Epithalamus*

(1) Applying acupuncture to ST 36 could produce the effect of analgesia through the regulation of the discharge of the "pain" excitement unit of the lateral habenular body (Fu *et al.*, 1983).

(2) Stimulating the habenular body could weaken the effect of acupuncture analgesia. If applying acupuncture could raise a large mouse's pain threshold, the use of L-glutamic acid to excite the habenular body could obviously lower the analgesia of acupuncture (Wang *et al.*, 1988).

(3) Using microelectrophoresis to supply Ach to the lateral habenular body, it was observed that Ach had an excitement function on the performance of most neuronal spontaneous discharges of the habenular body; a microdose injection of Ach in the habenular body could produce remarkable antagonist to EA analgesia (Pan *et al.*, 1997).

1.4 The Function of Brain Stem Structure in Acupuncture Analgesia

1.4.1 *Medulla oblongata*

(1) Using radioactive isotopes to mark deoxy-glucose, it was observed that in the application of acupuncture analgesia or stimulation of caudate nucleus, the metabolic rates of the anterior of medulla oblongata ventral gigantocellular reticular nucleus and the Nucleus Paraglgantocellularis Lateralis (PGCL) were apparently increased. This indicated that they positively took part in the process of acupuncture analgesia (Zhou *et al.*, 1991).

(2) Employing the glass electrode extracellular recording method, observations could be made on the change in discharge of a large mouse's neurons in its rostral ventromedial medulla (RVM). It was found that two frequencies of electrical acupuncture applied on acupoints, 2 and 10 Hz, could increase pain excited neurons' spontaneous discharge and inhibit their increased frequency response. The inhibited response from 2 Hz increased frequency could be completely blocked by Naloxone, but the response at 10 Hz could only be partially blocked by Naloxone (Ao *et al.*, 1996).

1.4.2 *Midbrain*

Inside the brain, the nucleus groups associated with analgesia mostly have fibers directly or indirectly projecting to Nucleus raphe magnus (NRM), through which they end up at the dorsal corner of the spinal cord. Applying electrophysiological technology, with the brain analgesia system mainly descending inhibition originated from NRM as the centre, a systematic study was conducted on the large mouse's cerebral cortex and some nucleus groups in terms of their regulation and control of NRM, together with their function in acupuncture analgesia.

(1) NRM neurons most of the time produced excitement, inhibition or transformation responses of excited inhibition under nociceptive stimulation. NRM could be activated by applying acupuncture to "ST 36" or other acupoints, of which nociceptive response come up with apparent analgesia. NRM neurons are regulated and controlled by cinerea, head of the caudate nucleus and nucleus accumbens. Stimulating these nucleus groups could activate NRM, inducing analgesia, while the lateral habenular body has a duplex function on NRM, causing excitement during stimulation and inhibition after stimulation has stopped. It was also found that when any of the nucleus groups was damaged, the function of acupuncture analgesia would weaken or disappear, even inducing an oversensitivity to pain (Liu, 1996).

(2) There were other experiments revealing that Red Nucleus (RN) of the midbrain also took part in the process of acupuncture analgesia. For example, both electrical stimulation of RN and acupuncture of "ST 36" would inhibit C response of neurons of the dorsal corner of the spinal cord; and electrical stimulation of RN could strengthen the analgesic effect of acupuncture. The use of Naloxone could reverse the inhibition effect of C response produced as a result of electrical stimulation of RN. The result is an indication that opiate system took part in the regulating function by RN in response to acupuncture analgesia (Han, 1988).

(3) The surrounding PAG of the central aqueduct is a key location of the intrinsic analgesia system. By injecting 5-HT receptor antagonist with a microdose of cinnamic thiamin into a domestic rabbit's PAG location, the basic pain threshold was not affected but analgesia was weakened. It was suggested that under the influence of acupuncture, 5-HT inside PAG could activate the synaptic transmission mechanism, inducing an analgesic effect (Kang *et al.*, 1983).

(4) There is one point that needs to be stressed: acupuncture analgesia can only achieve its greatest function and best therapeutic result subject to the condition that various structures inside the brain are intact, and with healthy functions (Liu, 1996).

1.5 The Spinal Cord in Acupuncture Analgesia

1.5.1 *Segmental inhibition of acupuncture analgesia involved both postsynaptic and pre-synaptic inhibitions*

Acupuncture analgesia on the spinal cord level has obvious segmental bearing; such an analgesic effect has the involvement of postsynaptic and pre-synaptic inhibitions. If acupuncture is applied to BL 32 and GB 30 of a mouse its tail-flick threshold could be raised. When acupuncture is applied to GB 30 of both sides (dorsal horn neurons) the nociceptive response of the dorsal neurons induced by sural nerve stimulation could be inhibited. Acupuncture applied to GB 34 could inhibit the nociceptive response induced by stimulation of dorsal horn neurons of the ankle; to PC 6 and HT 3 of the spinal cord of a cat (dorsal horn neurons), it could inhibit nociceptive response of dorsal horn neurons through the stimulation of thoracic sympathetic chain. Acupoints below any paraplegia level did not have any analgesic effect on pain control concerning splanchnic pain; the effect of paraplegia was so clear-cut, segmental mechanism used by acupuncture to inhibit pain of the skeletal parts is different from that of splanchnic pain. Intrathecal injection of Naloxone could block acupuncture from raising tail-flick threshold of a monkey. There was a case in which the spinal cord of a cat where acupuncture on bilateral GB 30 or ST 36 could inhibit nociceptive response of efferent neurons of the spinal dorsal horn and lengthen the latent period of reversed action potential. It follows that in segmental inhibition of acupuncture analgesia, both postsynaptic and presynaptic inhibitions are involved (Zhu *et al.*, 1989).

1.5.2 *The peripheral neurological structures related to acupuncture*

(1) A large number of experiments have proved that the peripheral transmission of acupuncture analgesic effect involve all four types of

fibers (I, II types of thick fibers and III, IV types of small fibers), of which the small fibers (III and IV) play a major role. If nociceptive acupuncture was applied to the proximity of sural nerve to induce a domestic rabbit's pain response due to mandibular reflex movement, while at the distal end of that nerve, supplying continuously electrical pulses to stimulate acupoints with a frequency of 5 Hz, observations on the analgesia effect of different types of nerve fibers could be conducted. The result indicated that in the course of acupuncture, the smaller the excitement fiber, the stronger the analgesia effect. It means that the effect of exciting fiber types I and II was smaller than exciting type III. The latter was again smaller than types I, II, III and IV together. A selective use of Novocain to block the transmission of small fibers (types III and IV) obviously weakened the analgesic effect, and shortened the continuity of time, indicating that when thick and small fibers were excited at the same time, the strengthening of analgesia was a result of the small fiber excitement, and not due to exciting more thick fibers. Concurrent with the increased intensity of electrical acupuncture, direct current of positive electrode was selectively used to block thick fibers, excite types III and IV alone, or simultaneously excite types III and IV fibers. Observations were made on analgesic effect of various fibers in terms of their descending sequence of strength: IV > III > I, II. In addition, the analgesic effects of simultaneously exciting types III and IV was greater than that by exciting types III or IV fibers alone. Using positive electrode of direct current to block the transmission of thick fibers, as a basis of observing the analgesic effects of small fibers, intravenous injection of Naloxone (0.4 mg/kg) was applied that could apparently cause the analgesic effect to weaken or even disappear. This indicated that the analgesic effect of small fibers has acupuncture analgesic effects features different from excitable analgesia (Tang *et al.*, 1989).

(2) It could be seen that electrical acupuncture analgesic effect is related to its frequencies. If a standard amount of electricity was used as a quantitative index for measuring different types of nerve fiber excitement, with reference to their transmission speeds, the change of electric potential range and course of time, a comprehensive analysis of

the influence of different frequency electrical acupuncture on different types of nerve fiber excitement could be made. Consequently, it was found that the electrical acupuncture frequency which can obviously lower excitement varies according to the type of nerve fiber involved. Type I fibers has the highest critical frequency rate (200 Hz), followed by type II fibers (100 Hz), with type III fibers still lower (10 Hz), while IV fibers has the lowest (5 Hz); however, following the increase of electrical frequency, the effect deepens continuously. For example, type I fibers at 1000 Hz, type II at 500 Hz, type III at 200 Hz and type IV at 20 Hz, after ten minutes of stimulation, their action electric potential would basically disappear, became residual or appear with double frequency, indicating that the nerve has fallen into a comparative non-responsive or fatigue state (Tang *et al.*, 1987).

(3) Recently, a lot of research has indicated that C fibers (that is, type IV fibers) have important impact in electrical acupuncture analgesia (Liu *et al.*, 1997). But others think that C fibers do not play an important role in acupuncture analgesia (Fan *et al.*, 1988). Some, however, think that C fibers are not the major fiber through which electrical acupuncture analgesia is transmitted. Rather the diffused nociceptive inhibited control fibers are mainly responsible (Bao *et al.*, 1991).

1.5.3 *Neurotransmitters related to acupuncture analgesia*

The central neurotransmitters have an important function on the process of acupuncture analgesia. Among the many central neurotransmitters four are most important for acupuncture: peptides, monoamines, amino acids and cholines.

Peptides

The peptide class of central neurotransmitter substances include many polypeptides, such as vasopressin, oxytocin, thyrotrophic releasing hormone (TRH), gonadotropin releasing hormone (GnRH), growth inhibitor, β-endorphin, enkephaline, dynorphin, and gastroenteric peptide, etc. In the course of acupuncture analgesia, the chief participants were endogenous opioid peptides (β-endorphin, enkephaline and dynorphin), primarily based on the following experimental evidence:

(1) Acupuncture promotes the release of opioid peptide substances. With the application of low frequency (2 Hz) electrical acupuncture, the release of methionine enkephalin (a kind of enkephaline) was increased, while with high frequency (100 Hz) EA the release of dynorphin A and B was increased; the poor effect of electrical acupuncture analgesia of mouse opioid peptide whose release has no apparent increase (Fei *et al.*, 1986). In an experiment to determine the amount of release of opioid peptide in the spinal subarachnoid perfusion under different frequencies of electrical acupuncture, it was found that high frequency electrical acupuncture mainly increased the dynorphic-like immunologically competent substance, whereas low frequency EA mainly increased methionine enkephalin-like immunologically competent substance (Han *et al.*, 1986). These results suggested that high frequency electrical acupuncture mainly facilitate spinal release of dynorphin and low frequency electrical acupuncture mainly facilitate spinal release of methionine enkephalin.

(2) Opioid peptide specific receptor blocker (such as Naloxone and Opioid Peptide antiserum) and agonist both can influence the analgesic effect of acupuncture. An injection of microdose of morphine receptor blocker, Naloxone, to nucleus accumbens and head of caudate nucleus could block analgesic effect of acupoint ST 36 by electrical acupuncture; when Naloxone was injected into the gray substance surrounding the aqueduct, it could not only block analgesic effect produced by electrical acupuncture on ST 36, but also that of morphine injection of the abdominal cavity, and furthermore, it could block the analgesic effect induced by the activation of Nucleus raphe magnus (NRM), resulting from the stimulation of nucleus accumbens and caudate nucleus. It is indicative that the endogenous morphine substance was the major transmitter for these analgesic structures participating in electrical acupuncture analgesia (Liu, 1996). Low frequency (2 Hz) electrical acupuncture analgesia could be blocked by only a small dose (0.5 mg/kg) of Naloxone while a higher dose

(20 mg/kg) was required to block high frequency (100 Hz) electrical acupuncture analgesia (Han *et al.*, 1986).

After an intrathecal injection of opioid peptide antiserum, observation could be made on its influence on the effect of electrical acupuncture analgesia. It was found that a FQ antiserum could selectively block 2 Hz electrical acupuncture analgesia, while dynorphin antiserum could selectively block 100 Hz electrical acupuncture analgesic effect (Xie *et al.*, 1985).

Using specific opiate receptor blocker and cross-tolerance method, a mechanism was worked out for 2–15 Hz electrical acupuncture analgesia of spinal bone receptor. It was found that in the course of applying 2-15 Hz electrical acupuncture, the release of endogenous opiate substance by the mouse spinal cord concurrently activated μ, δ, and κ, types of opiate receptors, of which the analgesic effect produced by 2–15 Hz electrical acupuncture depended on the coordinated function of these three types of opiate receptors. Blocking any one type of receptor could lead to the collapse of the whole coordinated function (Chen *et al.*, 1992).

Further research in the application of cross-tolerance and receptor blockage method found that high and low frequencies electrical acupuncture analgesia could be respectively blocked by δ and κ types of opiate blockers, while there was no cross-tolerance in high and low frequencies electrical acupuncture analgesia (Fei *et al.*, 1988). The injection of opiate receptor σ agonist Ketamine (with antagonist effect on opiate receptor type μ) could antagonize the analgesic effect produced by electrical acupuncture on unilateral LI 4 and TE 5 acupoints of domestic rabbit, while the combination of opiate receptor μ type agonist Fentanyl and DA receptor antagonist could strengthen and lengthen electrical acupuncture analgesic effect (Zhou *et al.*, 1985).

(3) Endogenous opiate substance (such as Cholecystokinin (CCK) reduce electrical acupuncture analgesic effect. If electrical acupuncture analgesia had no or very weak effect on a mouse, with antigen injection to its spinal subarachnoid after which electrical acupuncture was applied, an analgesic effect would appear (Han, 1988). In other experiments, it was found when electrical acupuncture was applied for too long, it would weaken the analgesic effect, and the result could

be related to the release of Cholecystokinin (CCK-8). If electrical acupuncture was applied continuously to the mouse for more than two hours, the content of CCK-8 in Central Spinal Fluid (CSF) was obviously raised, indicating the accelerated release of CCK-8; the content of CCK-8 in Periaqueductal gray (PAG) surrounding aqueduct of the midbrain was also increasing, indicating that the processing of CCK precursor in producing CCK-8 has been accelerated. With electrical acupuncture lasting for eight hours, mRNA level of CCK in the brain was found to be significantly elevated, indicating the gene transcription has speeded up, while CCK-8 antigen inverted the electrical acupuncture tolerance. The electrical acupuncture tolerance caused by a continuous electrical acupuncture application for six hours could be inverted by the injection of CCK antiserum in ventricle; and the use of CCK receptor antagonist would strengthen electrical acupuncture analgesia, preventing electrical acupuncture tolerance. CCK receptor antagonist could strengthen high frequency (100 Hz) electrical acupuncture analgesic effect, whereas low frequency (2 Hz) electrical acupuncture did not have such effect. The CCK_A antagonist Devazepide and CCK_B receptor antagonist could delay the appearance of electrical acupuncture tolerance; however, the function of CCK_B receptor antagonist was obviously stronger than that of CCK_A, indicating that the effect of CCK was mainly achieved through B type of receptor. In the experiment, it was also found that applying electrical acupuncture to the mouse for 30 min could elevate the concentration of CCK-8 in spinal perfusion for which 15 Hz and 100 Hz electrical acupuncture had higher function than that of 2 Hz (Zhou *et al.*, 1993). If electrical acupuncture was applied continuously for six hours, CCK-8 in CSF would also be maintained at a high level. Upon lengthening the electrical acupuncture time for 2–3 hours without break, the content of CCK-8 in the brain was found to be obviously elevated, which dropped down after four hours; in eight hours CCK mRNA content was found to be obviously elevated, indicating the synthesis was accelerated (Han, 2000; Sun *et al.*, 1995; Zhou *et al.*, 1993).

(4) The opiate system might take part in the process of peripheral analgesia. On the inflammatory spot, a small amount of injected Naloxone could block the electrical acupuncture analgesic effect, suggesting that

acupuncture could possibly provoke the inflammatory area to release endo-opioid peptide whose function on opiate receptor is sensitized by inflammation, leading to the inflammatory area to produce stronger electrical acupuncture analgesic effect (Zhu, 1993).

Among the endogenous opiate peptide substances, there is yet one more kind, Orphanin FQ, for which experimental research found that FQ could weaken electrical acupuncture analgesic effect. If the lateral ventricle of cerebrum was injected with FQ, it could weaken electrical acupuncture analgesia, whereas the same place was injected with FQ antibody would strengthen EA analgesia (Tian *et al.*, 2000). Applying electrical acupuncture to a mouse's unilateral "GB 30" and "GB 34" acupoints, midbrain Ventrolateral periaquedutal gray (VPAG) surrounding the aqueduct, Dorsal Raphe Nucleus (DRN), NRM nucleus groups FQ receptor mRNA indicated an apparent drop, suggesting that FQ inside the brain and its receptor could both possibly take part in the process of acupuncture analgesia (Ma *et al.*, 2004).

Substance P is closely related to pain sense. On the spinal cord level, it takes the function of transmitting pain sense signal, while on the brainstem level, the analgesic function. Some research found that substance P and EA analgesia could have a coordinating function, strengthening EA analgesic effects (Zhang *et al.*, 1980b).

Monoamines

In the study of acupuncture analgesia, the related monoamine class of central nervous transmitters mainly includes 5-hydroxytryptamine (5-HT), dopamine and noradrenalin.

(1) 5-hydroxytryptamine (5-HT). There is no consensus on the influence of acupuncture on the 5-HT content in the brain. Some reported that after acupuncture on locations such as the diencephalon, there was an increase in 5-HT content, while some reported that after acupuncture, there was no change in the content of 5-HT in the brain. The appearance of such results could possibly due to the fact that the media in the body were subject to constant updating process. Just simply measuring the content of certain media could not fully reflect the important

meaning of its physiological function. As such, some researchers have injected p-Chlorophenylalanine (pCPA) into the ventricle of the domestic rabbit, aimed at a selective inhibition of tryptophan hydroxylase and lowering of the content of 5-HT (with less effect on other monoamine class media) in the brain, in a study of the content of 5-HT in the brain in response to acupuncture. In the domestic rabbit, after injecting pCPA into the ventricle of the brain, the diencephalon, lower brain stem and cerebral cortex showed lower contents of 5-HT than in the controlled group, by 79.2%, 48.5% and 9.6% respectively. Concurrently, the analgesic effect by finger needling, electrical acupuncture and morphine were obviously lower, suggesting that the intensity of acupuncture analgesic effect was closely related to the content of 5-HT in the diencephalon and the lower brain stem (Beijing Medical College research group on fundamental theory acupuncture anesthesia, 1975a). After two months, using the same animal whose 5-HT has recovered naturally, or were injected with 5-Hydroxy tryptophan (5-HTP) to speed up 5-HT elevation, it was found that the acupuncture analgesic effect has also recovered. When a normal mouse was injected with 5-HTP to induce a high increase in 5-HT content in the brain, acupuncture analgesic effect was obviously strengthened (Beijing Medical College research group on fundamental theory of acupuncture anesthesia, 1978a).

In another group of experiment using rats, the mouse was injected with Pargyline, a monoamine oxidase inhibitor which raises 5-HT content in the brain, strengthen the Electro-Acupuncture (EA) analgesic effect on the rats (Beijing Medical College research group on fundamental theory of acupuncture anesthesia, 1975b).

To further explore the descending and ascending pathways of 5-HT in solution to its function in acupuncture analgesia, 5,6-dihydroxytryptamine (DHT) (a kind of 5-HT related chemical blocker of nerve fibers) was injected into a mouse's brain ventricle, to destroy 5-HT that is descending from the brain stem NRM group to the spinal cord. It was found that it selectively blocked those 5-HT ascending fibers. DHT lowered the 5-HT content of the spinal cord by 66–83%, but there was no sign of weakening in the acupuncture analgesic effects. When the medial forebrain bundle (lateral hypothalamus area) or dorsal raphe nucleus and median nucleus ascending fibers were injected with DHT at their afferent ends, the 5-HT content of the forebrain dropped by 52%, while there was no apparent effect on the 5-HT content of spinal cord, then the EA analgesic effect was obviously lowered. The results suggested that 5-HT ascending fibers from the brain stem median nucleus group going forward to the forebrain had an important impact on acupuncture analgesia (Beijing Medical College fundamental group on the theory of acupuncture anesthesia, 1978b).

To explain in the course of EA analgesia what happens in the dynamic changing process of 5-HT metabolism, an experiment was conducted on the influence of EA on the contents of 5-HT in a mouse's brain and spinal cord, applying at the same time two drugs, Pargyline and Probenecid. The renewal rate of central 5-HT was found that (1) under the influence of EA, the synthesis and use of central 5-HT were both speeded up, however, synthesis outstripped usage, resulting in the increase of content; (2) with reference to the speed of synthesis, that for the spinal cord and brain stem increased, and with regard to the speed of forebrain endbrain and diencephalon increased, suggesting that forebrain 5-HT in acupuncture analgesia could be functionally more important; and (3) EA stimulation had no obvious influence on the speed of eliminating metabolic product by central 5-HT (Beijing Medical College fundamental research group on the theory of acupuncture and anesthesia, 1978c).

There were other experiments which indicated that acupuncture analgesic effect is related to the level of 5-HT content in the brain induced by acupuncture. If Levotryotophan (100 or 200 mg/kg) was injected into a mouse's abdominal cavity, it could increase 5-HT content in the brain by 22% and 31% respectively, without any obvious influence on EA analgesic effect. However, when the abdominal cavity was injected with more than 60 mg/kg of 5-HTP, it doubled the 5-HT content in the mouse brain, subsequently strengthening the EA analgesia (Beijing Medical College fundamental research group on the theory of acupuncture and anesthesia, 1978d). The results suggested that the production of analgesic effect by EA was related to the increase of 5-HT content level in the brain.

(2) Dopamine (DA). After the rats' frontal part of the caudate nucleus was damaged by means of electrolysis method, the acupuncture analgesic effect was obviously lowered. However when the damage occurred in the central area, the needling effect was apparently increased, suggesting that under biological conditions, the frontal part of caudate nucleus has the function of facilitating the acupuncture analgesic effect, while the central area has inhibited function. After injecting 6-hydroxy dopamine (6-OH-DA) into the frontal or central area, the change in acupuncture analgesic effect was opposite to the result of electrical damage, suggesting that on the one hand, different areas of the caudate nucleus exerted different influences on the acupuncture analgesic effect, while on the other, it explained that messages transmitted by the dopaminergic fibers could be responsible. It leads to the belief that acupuncture message could be transmitted to caudate nucleus through non-dopaminergic fibers (Zhang *et al.*, 1978).

To clarify the dopamine receptor effects from different nuclear groups in EA, it was observed that nucleus accumbens and caudate nucleus have strong influence (Wang *et al.*, 1997).

The caudate nucleus is the largest basal nucleus in the brain. It was generally considered as primarily related to motor regulation and control, however, later research found that caudate nucleus was also related to sensory mechanism and it could affect the sensory transmission activity. Needling the acupoints of the Governor Vessel of a domestic rabbit would cause an obvious increase of the contents of brain caudate nucleus 3–4 dopamine and HVA, its major ultimate metabolic products. When the dorsolateral head of caudate nucleus of the domestic rabbit was damaged, acupuncture analgesic effect was apparently lowered, indicating dopamine neuron activity was strengthened and that the caudate nucleus dopamine level in the process of producing acupuncture effect could have an important function (Feng *et al.*, 1978).

When a domestic rabbit was given intravenous and brain ventricle injections of reserpine (1 mg/kg, 0.25 mg/kg) after 24 hours, EA effect was obviously strengthened. Based on this fact, the domestic rabbit was again given celiac injection of L-DOPA of catecholamine (100 mg/kg), restoring part of the content of catecholamine in the brain. It was found that the analgesic effect was apparently lowered or basically disappeared, a sign further indicating that central reserpine could antagonize EA. The experiment also found that reserpine has influence in strengthening morphine analgesia, suggesting that acupuncture analgesia and morphine analgesia could have different principles (Beijing Medical College fundamental research group on the theory of acupuncture and anesthesia, 1978e).

(3) Noradrenalin. When a domestic rabbit's cerebral ventricle is injected with piperidine or phentolamine, the central dopamine receptor or adrenergic α receptor is blocked, leading to the strengthening of acupuncture analgesia. On the other hand, when the cerebral ventricle was injected with morphine or clonidine hydrochloride, the central dopamine receptor and β receptor were excited, thereby causing significant weakening of acupuncture analgesia. If the cerebral ventricle was injected with β receptor blocker, propanolol, or β receptor agonist, isoproterenol, there was no obvious influence on acupuncture analgesic. The experimental results suggested that central catecholamines have a counter actual function on acupuncture analgesia (Beijing Medical College fundamental research group on the theory of acupuncture anesthesia, 1978f). Injection of noradrenaline in the abdominal cavity has no effect on central α receptors because of the blood-brain barrier. It was suggested that the central α receptors, when excited, have antagonizing effects on acupuncture analgesia (Beijing Medical College fundamental research group on the theory of acupuncture and anesthesia, 1978g).

6-hydroxydopamine (6-OHDA) is a chemical blocker of catecholaminergic nerve fibers. It was found that an injection of 6-OHDA into the ventricular girdle of the brain for 48 hours, while norepinephrine level in the brain is lowered, appears to strengthen EA effects, suggesting that norepinephrine ascending fibers in the brain could have a counter effect to EA (Beijing Medical College fundamental research on the theory of acupuncture and anesthesia, 1978h). After injection of 6-OHDA was made in the medulla to damage the noradrenalinergic neurons descending path, it was found that the animal's EA becomes apparently weakened, suggesting that noradrenalinergic descending system could strengthen EA function (Ye *et al.*, 1982). It should be noted that noradrenalinergic neuronal system in acupuncture analgesia has bidirectional functions.

1.5.4 *The regulative pathways of acupuncture analgesia*

The "Gate-control" theory

The "gate-control" theory was put forward by Melzack and Wall in 1965, and aims at explaining the segmental regulating function of pain by the spinal cord. The theory believes that segmental regulation of neural network is formed by primary afferent A δ and C fibers, dorsal horn projecting neurons (T cells), and glial area inhibitive intermediate nerve (SG cells), in which afferent A δ and C fibers could both activate the activity of T cells. Their function on Substantia Gelatinosa (SG) cells is just the opposite in that the primary afferent A δ fibers could excite SG cells while afferent C fibers could inhibit SG cells. Thus, peripheral nociceptive stimulation excites C fibers of which afferent tonic activity makes the gate open, allowing nociceptive message to transmit via T cells to higher centers, producing the sensation of pain. When there is some contact, rubbing, massaging or stimulation which excites A type afferent fibers, making SG cells excited, thereby closing the gate, inhibiting T cells activity, thus preventing or cutting down nociceptive message from transmitting to higher centre, resulting in pain relief. Afterwards, in 1983, proponents of the "gate theory" revised and supplemented their original theory: (1) emphasizing the multifunction of SG cells, which has both inhibitive and exciting functions; the gate's prohibitive pattern on T cells can be either presynaptic or postsynaptic; and (2) emphasizing the function of descending prohibitive system of the reticular formation of the brainstem, and this kind of inhibition is only afferent to the gate (Qin *et al.*, 1985).

Applying "gate theory" to explain the mechanism of acupuncture analgesia, it is generally believed that the stimulation message procedure by acupuncture is transmitted by the thick fibers, which prevents the conduction of nociceptive stimulation, resulting in analgesic effect. This could explain part of the mechanism of acupuncture analgesia. But in reality, as indicated by most of research materials cited recently, in the course of acupuncture analgesia, the analgesic effect of C fibers excels that of A fibers, which can hardly be explained by gate theory. Yet the supplementary materials of "gate theory", in which the descending inhibitive system of reticular formation of the brainstem, inhibitive pattern of the gate on T cells — presynaptic inhibition and postsynaptic inhibition, etc. — could all be verified in recent research on the mechanism of acupuncture analgesia.

Thalamic nucleus submedius

An artificially damaged thalamic nucleus submedius (Sm) facilitates its nociceptive behavioral response. On the other hand, electro or chemical stimulation of Sm or Ventrolateral orbital (VLO) cortex inhibits the response of nociceptic behaviour and the spinal cord dorsal horn neurons nociceptic response. Studies showed that these responses could be cancelled by damaging VLO the aqueduct. Nociceptic stimulation and hand needling stimulation could activate Sm neurons activity. When the Sm or VLO was damaged, it would weaken the analgesia of excited small fibers caused by strong EA, but there was no apparent influence on weak EA function. These effects could respectively be blocked by each of their receptor antagonists. When Sm or VLO was subjected to intra-injection of GABA, it could quickly weaken morphine or 5-HT induced inhibition; whereas injecting GABA receptor antagonist, bicuculline, inhibited the response of nociceptic behaviour and strengthened morphine and 5-HT induced inhibition. It was inferred that in the central nervous system, there is a pain sense regulated negative feedback loop, formed by spinal cord-Sm-VLO-PAG-spinal cord, which plays an important function in analgesia produced by excited small fibers under acupuncture (Tang *et al.*, 2002).

1.6 The Relationship between EA Function and Stimulation Parameter

1.6.1 *Influence of frequency and waveform on the effect of acupuncture anesthesia in EA*

A study on 226 patients who were receiving birth control operations, using acupuncture anesthesia of different combination of acupoints was completed, and the results revealed that under the same strength of acupuncture and waveform, with high frequency the effect of anesthesia of needling next to the incision was better than with lower frequency. The most steady effect was found at frequency 800 Hz, at all stages of the operation. The effect of anesthesia is loose and compact waveforms.

1.6.2 *Influence of voltage on the effect of analgesia*

With a stimulation frequency rate of 100 times/min and under the condition of continuous waveform, a comparison was made on different stimulation strengths that affect the analgesic effect of a normal person. (1) Unchanged peak voltage: within 25 minutes from the beginning of needling until the end, there was no change in the peak voltage, maintaining at 1 V. (2) Changing peak voltage once: at the beginning of the needling, peak voltage was 1 V and after 10 minutes, peak voltage was raised to 2 V, changing only once. (3) Gradual change of peak voltage: needling started with voltage of 1 V, in 5 mins voltage was raised to 1.5 V, 10 mins 2.0 V, 15 mins 2.5 V and 20 mins 3.0 V. Results indicated that whether the peak voltage change once does not change, there was no apparent difference in EA effect. The effect of gradual change in the voltage was apparently better than steady voltage (Zhang *et al.*, 1979).

1.6.3 *Influence of wave width on the effect of anesthesia*

An EA stimulation experiment was conducted on a domestic rabbit, applying acupuncture anesthesia on the side of the spine and using dual direction matrix wave through a dual directional stimulator. Frequency rate was set at 60 Hz, and observations were made on different wave widths (0.05, 0.1, 0.5, 1.0, 2.5, 5.0, 8.0 ms respectively) and their impacts on the effect of EA anesthesia. It was found that when the frequency rate was fixed at 60 Hz, electrical current strength set at 1 mA, as wave width was narrowed and peak voltage value was increased, the corresponding pain threshold of the animal was apparently raised, but the animal showed unrest and discomfort, suggesting that the raised pain threshold failed to satisfy the need. When the frequency rate was fixed at 60 Hz, and strength of stimulation was increased gradually, different wave widths could put the animal under anesthesia, but the 1 ms wave width group achieved the best results when the animal remained calm. This suggested that electrical current and voltage, at their lowest value of combined action, produced better acupuncture anesthesia effect.

1.6.4 *Influence of EA frequency rate and position on analgesic effect*

Studies had been conducted to compare the analgesic effect of different afferent fibers of distal and near segments, and under high or low frequencies (high frequency being 100 Hz and low one at 5 Hz). It was discovered that irrespective of distant or near segments, high or low frequencies, the basic performance of EA was: the smaller the fibers, the stronger the analgesic effect. Using low frequency EA stimulating type I, II and III fibers, the analgesic function was greater than those of the high frequencies. In the distant segment, there was no such difference between the high low frequencies stimulation. Stimulating the near segment with high frequency and distant segment with low frequency stimulation, it appeared that different degrees of adaptation would occur (Wang *et al.*, 1982).

1.7 Conclusion

Summarizing the above, it should be noted that acupuncture analgesia is produced through the stimulation of needling (including EA), which induces change in the mechanism of pain perception, from peripheral to different levels of the central nervous system, involving nerves, body fluids humoral and many other factors, sensitize or nullify pain, separately or jointly in a double complex dynamic processes. In these processes, the function of nervous system and the neurotransmission are working simultaneously. A lot of research findings have proved the objectivity of acupuncture analgesia, resulting in widespread application and further research. Yet there are still many unknown facts and uncertainties in acupuncture analgesia. The important uncertainties include: the unsteady therapeutic effect; the individual differences; the divergent needling techniques; the room for optimization; the selection of acupoints; and the difficulties in the evaluation. Regardless of many clinical and animal studies, there is yet no uniform and precise test for pain assessment.

Providing analgesia is one of the important challenges in medicine. The effect of acupuncture analgesia is beyond doubt, and it is one of the cheapest therapeutic means that does not use medication, has very little side effects, and commands much diversities. With its rising popularity, it is important for scientists to work closely with clinicians so that acupuncture effects could be better ensured and more repeatable for patients suffering from pain.

References

Acupuncture anesthesia Principle Research Seminar, Peking Medical College Fundamentals Department. (1975a) Central nervous media's role in acupuncture analgesia. I. Chlorophenyl alanine acupuncture analgesia in rabbits. *Chin. Sci. Bull.* **10**, 483–485.

Acupuncture anesthesia Principle Research Seminar, Peking Medical College Fundamentals Department. (1975b) Central nervous media's role in acupuncture analgesia. II. Pargyline on electroacupuncture analgesia in rabbits. *Chin. Sci. Bull.* **11**, 532–534.

Acupuncture anesthesia Principle Research Seminar, Peking Medical College Fundamentals Department. (1976) Central nervous media's role in acupuncture analgesia. V. Chlorophenyl alanine and 5-hydroxytryptophan on acupuncture analgesia in rats. *J. Peking Univ, (Health Sci.)* **4**, 224–228, 233.

Acupuncture anesthesia Principle Research Seminar, Peking Medical College Fundamentals Department. (1978a) The role of central nervous media in acupuncture analgesia. VII. Intraventricular and intracerebral injection of 5,6-HT on electroacupuncture analgesia in rats. *Acupunct. Res.* **1**, 46.

Acupuncture anesthesia Principle Research Seminar, Peking Medical College Fundamentals Department. (1978b) The role of central nervous media in acupuncture analgesia. VIII the study of electroacupuncture analgesia on the process of central 5-hydroxytryptamine update rate in rats. *Acupunct. Res.* **1**, 47.

Acupuncture anesthesia Principle Research Seminar, Peking Medical College Fundamentals Department. (1978c) The role of central nervous media in acupuncture analgesia. VI. Tryptophan and 5-hydroxytryptophan on the electro-acupuncture analgesia in rat. *Acupunct. Res.* **1**, 45–46.

Acupuncture anesthesia Principle Research Seminar, Peking Medical College Fundamentals Department. (1978d) The role of central nervous media in acupuncture analgesia. IX Effects of electro-acupuncture and noxious stimuli on unit discharge of dorsal raphe nuclear of rat. *Acupunct. Res.* **1**, 48.

Acupuncture anesthesia Principle Research Seminar, Peking Medical College Fundamentals Department. (1978e) The role of central nervous media in acupuncture analgesia XI reserpine and DOPA affect on acupuncture analgesia and morphine analgesia in rabbits. *Acupunct. Res.* **1**, 49–50.

Acupuncture anesthesia Principle Research Seminar, Peking Medical College Fundamentals Department. (1978f) The role of central nervous media in acupuncture analgesia V intraventricular injection of catecholamine receptor blocking agents and agonists on the analgesic effect of rabbit. *Acupunct. Res.* **1**, 49.

Acupuncture anesthesia Principle Research Seminar, Peking Medical College Fundamentals Department. (1978g) The role of central nervous media in acupuncture analgesia.

XVI the clonidine and phentolamine effects on electroacupuncture analgesia in rats. *Acupunct. Res.* **1**, 54.

Acupuncture anesthesia Principle Research Seminar, Peking Medical College Fundamentals Department. (1878h) The role of central nervous media in acupuncture analgesia XVII. 6-OHDA lesions of the rat brain noradrenergic uplink fiber affecting on electroacupuncture analgesia. *Acupunct. Res.* **1**, 54–55.

Ao, M., Wei, J., Tan, Z., *et al.* (1996) The influence of electroacupuncture with different frequencies on the discharges of neurons in rostral ventromedial medulla on rats. *Acupunct. Res.* **4**, 41–45.

Bao, H., Zhou, Z. and Yu, Y. (1991) C fiber is not necessary in electroacupuncture analgesia, but necessary in diffuse noxious inhibitory controls (DNIC). *Acupunct. Res.* **16**(2), 120–124.

Cao, X., Xu, S., He, L., *et al.* (1989) Acupuncture activates pain modulating system resulting in acupuncture analgesia. *Acupunct. Res.* **1–2**, 199–200.

Chen, Z., Weng, J., Ren, H., *et al.* (1980) The relationship of cerebral cortex and acupuncture inhibition of visceral pain I. Effects of electro-acupuncture on the greater splanchnic nerve. *J. Sun Yat-sen Univ. (Med. Sci.)* **1**(1), 1–8.

Chen, X., Kang, M., Zhao, C., *et al.* (1992) The three types of opioid receptors in the rat spinal cord involved in the 2–15Hz electroacupuncture analgesia. *J. Beijing Univ. Tradit. Chin. Med.* **24**(1), 54.

Fan, S., Xie, X. and Han, J. (1988) Using of capsaicin to study the afferent fiber composition of electroacupuncture analgesia. *Chin. Sci. Bull.* **33**(17), 135.

Fei, H., Sun, S. and Han, J. (1988) Some evidences of supporting high-frequency and low frequency electro-acupuncture to release dynorphin and enkephalin in the spinal cord. *Chin. Sci. Bull.* **9**, 703–706.

Fei, H., Xie. G. and Han, J. (1986) Different frequency of electro-acupuncture analgesic effect is related to the release of spinal cord enkephalin and dynorphin. *Chin. Sci. Bull.* **19**, 1512–1515.

Feng, X., Ye, W., Zhao, D., *et al.* (1978) EA rabbit "Du Mai" points on the caudate nucleus of dopamine and its metabolites. *Chin. Sci. Bull.* **23**(5), 314–315.

Fu, Q., Fu, J. and Wang, S. (1983) Effect of acupuncture point on the discharges of "pain" units in lateral habenular nuclei (LH). *Acupunct. Res.* **4**, 262–265.

Han, J., Ding, X. and Fan, S (1986) The extent of the opioid receptor antagonist flip electroacupuncture analgesia dependent on the frequency of electroacupuncture. *Acta Physiologica Sinica* **38**(5), 475–482.

Han, J. (1988) Recent progress in the study of acupuncture mechanisms. *Acupunct. Res.* **1**, 36–38.

Han, J. (2000) Effect of anti-opioid of central cholecystokinin octapeptide is an important factor in determining the effectiveness of acupuncture analgesia and morphine analgesia. *Prog. Physiolo. Sci.* **31**(2), 173–177.

Kang, B., Zhou, Z. and Han, J. (1983) The periaqueductal gray 5-serotonin receptors of rabbits are involved in electroacupuncture analgesia and morphine analgesia. *Chin. Sci. Bull.* **14**, 888–891.

Liu, X., Huang, P. and Jiang, M. (1997) The effects of capsaicin blocking C fibers of nervi peroneus communis and its influence on analgesia of EA at "Zusanli". *Acupunct. Res.* **22**(4), 295–303.

Liu, X. (1996) The modulation of cerebral cortex and subcortical nucleion NRM and their role in acupuncture analgesia. *Acupunct. Res.* **21**(1), 4–11.

Ma, F., Xie, H., Dong, Z., *et al.* (2004) Effect of electroacupuncture on expression of ORL_1 receptor mRNA in some brain nuclei of the neuropathic pain rats. *Shanghai J. Acupunct. Moxibustion* **23**(4), 32–36.

Pan, Y, Wu, J. and Wang, S. (1997) Acetylcholine (Ach) excited the lateral habenula nucleus antagonistic electroacupuncture analgesia. *Acad. Period. Changchun Coll. Tradit. Chin. Med.* **13**(61), 58–59.

Qin, C. and Zhu, H. (1985) The new modification and evaluation of pain gate control theory. *Foreign Med. Anesthesiol. Resusc.* **4**, 160–161.

Sun, Y-H., Zhou, Y., Zhang, Z-W., *et al.* (1995) Accelerated release and production of CCK-8 in central nervous system of rats during prolonged electroacupuncture. *Chin. J. Neurosci.* **2**(2), 83–88.

Tang, J., Shi, W. and Hou, Z. (1987) Effects of electoracupuncture stimulation (eas) of different frequencies on the extitability of fibres of various groups. *Acupunct. Res.* **1**, 68–73.

Tang, J. and Yuan, B. (1989) The research on afferent fibers of acupuncture analgesia. *Acupunct. Res.* **14**(1–2), 135.

Tang, J. and Yuan, B. (2002) Discovery of a new pain modulation pathway. *J. Xi'an Jiaotong Univ. (Med.)* **23**(4), 329–332.

Tian, J.H. and Han, J.S. (2000) Functional studies using antibodies against orphanin FQ/ nociceptin. *Peptides* **21**(7), 1047–1050.

Wang, S., Gao, Y., Liu, G., *et al.* (1988) Effects of habenular nucleus and arcuate nucleus on pain threshold and acupuncture analgesia in rats. *Chin. J. Appl. Physiol.* **4**, 313.

Wang, Y., Feng, H., Cao, X., *et al.* (1997) Relation between electroacupuncture analgesia and dopamine receptors in nucleus accumbens and nucleus caudate. *Acupunct. Res.* **1–2**, 32.

Wang, Y., Yuan, Y. and Tang, J. (2006) Different-intensity electroacupuncture at thalamic nucleus submedius for analgesic effects. *Chin. J. Clin. Rehabil.* **10**(27), 38–41.

Wang, J., Tang, J., Hu A., *et al.* (1982) Comparison of different distance segments and low and high-frequency electro-acupuncture excitement through various types of afferent nerve fibers on analgesic effects. *Curr. Zoolog.* **28**(2), 136–140.

Wu, GJ., Chen, ZQ. and Shi, H. (2002) Roles of globus pallidus in acupuncture analgesia and exciting caudate-putamen nucleus-induced analgesia. *Chin. J. Neurosci.* **18**(3), 621–625.

Xie, G. and Han, J. (1985) Dynorphin B to enhance the analgesic effect of dynorphin A in the spinal cord. *Chin. Sci. Bull.* **15**, 1189–1191.

Xu, W., Yan, Y. and Chen, Z. (1989) Effects of Electroacupuncture on nociceptive responses observed on different days after lesion of unilateral somatosensory corted. *Acupunct. Res.* **4**, 424–427.

Xu, W., Gao, H. and Ye, Y. (1980) A study of the role of the cerebral cortex in acupuncture analgesia by the method of operant conditioning. *Acupunct. Res.* **4**, 268–273.

Xu, W., Lin, Y. and Zhang, Y. (1984) Active effects of the electro-acupuncture on the area of somatosensory neurons of the cerebral cortex. *Sci. Physiol.* **4**(5–6), 87.

Yang, J., Qu, Y. and Jia, H. (2001) Responses of neurons in the thalamic nucleus submedius to different stimulation in the rat. *J. Yanan Univ. (Nat. Sci. Ed.)* **20**(4), 61–64.

Ye, W., Dong, X., Jiang, Z., *et al.* (1982) Effect of intracerebral injection of 6-hydroxy-dopamine on the electro-acupuncture analgesic in rat. *Chin. Sci. Bull.* **13**, 821–824.

Zhang, C., Ye, L., Wang, H., *et al.* (1980) Analgesic effect of Substance P into the raphe nuclei on acupuncture analgesia. *J. Guiyang Med. Coll.* **5**(1), 29–35.

Zhang, D., Gu, X., San, H., *et al.* (1978) The stimulating and suppression of acupuncture analgesia responding to different regions of rat head of caudate nucleus. *Acta Physiologica Sinica* **30**(1), 21–28.

Zhang, J. and Wang, J. (1979) The relationship of electrical stimulation parameters and acupuncture anesthesia effect. *Acupunct. Res.* **1**, 1–7.

Zhang, J., Weng, J., Chen, P., *et al.* (1980) The relationship of cerebral cortex and acupuncture inhibition of visceral pain III. "Neiguan" cortical projection area and its impact on the discharge of cortical visceral pain. *J. Sun Yat-sen Univ. (Med. Sci.)* **1**(3), 253–258.

Zhou, Y., Sun, Y.H. and Han, J.S. (1993) Increased release of immunoreactive CCK-8 by electroacupuncture and enhancement of eectroacupuncture analgesia by CCK-8 Antagonist in rat spinal cord. *Neuropeptides* **24**, 139–144.

Zhou, Y., Li, Y. and Xu, S. (1985) Effect on Opiate Agonists on Acupuncture Analgesia. *J. Shanghai Med. Univ.* **12**(3), 219–232.

Zhou, J., Tian, Q, Hu, Z., *et al.* (1991) Morphological basis for brain and acupuncture stimulating produced analgesia 3–4 studies on rostroventral medulla in rat. *Acupunct. Res.* **z1**, 162.

Zhu, L., Fang, ZR, Li, C., *et al.* (1989) The role of segmental inhibition in acupuncture analgesia (AA). *Acupunct. Res.* **14**(1–2), 90–91.

Zhu, L., Li, C., Ji, C., *et al.* (1993) The role of OLS in peripheral acupuncture analgesia in arthritic rats. *Acupunct. Res.* **8**(3), 214–218.

Chapter 2

Acupuncture for Neurological Deficits

Abstract

Acupuncture theories suggest that the meridians link up viscera, organs, limbs and the different orifices through longitudinal channels to form an organic whole. The meridian concept is an important supporting principle in Chinese Medicine. The meridians largely follow the peripheral nervous system so that one of the modern explanations given to acupuncture is the assumption that the puncturing messages travel along the peripheral nerves, either directly or along closely related channels. The functional relationship is expressed on different levels: from the cerebral cortex, diencephalon, middle brain, brain stem, cerebellum, medulla oblongata, spinal chord to the peripheral nerves, running along both cephalic and caudal directions. While the neurological theory serves to give an easy explanation, the meridian system of acupuncture is far more complicated. Hidden and unexplained pathways are evident when acupuncture initiates exiting restorations of neurological deficits.

This chapter will give a brief account of the influence of acupuncture on neurological deficits.

Keywords: Meridian System; Nervous System; Cerebral Function.

2.1 Influence of Acupuncture on Cerebral Function

2.1.1 *Motor evoked potential (MEP)*

When acupuncture is applied corresponding to the cerebral cortex motor area to the scalp projecting area of a healthy person or a patient suffering from central nervous disease dyskinesia, it is possible to record the motor evoked potential (MEP) at the short abductor muscle of thumb, together with the latent period involved, and the post-needling effect. When the acupuncture MEP is compared with the MEP from direct trancranial electrical stimulation and magnetic stimulation, they were found to be basically the same in terms of waveform and duration, except that the amplitude voltage is smaller (μV). Another discovery is that while stimulation of the morbid lateral hemisphere could not initiate the MEP of contralateral hand muscles, when stimulating the contralateral lesion, MEP response was detected in some patients' ipsilateral hand muscles. It was inferred that the mechanical stimulation of the acupuncture motor area of the scalp could have turned on some sort of bioelectrical message in the cortex, passing through a certain afferent pathway, to excite the motor cortical neurons or fibers, which produced motor potential and again was transmitted to the descending motor transmission system, reaching the corresponding muscles (Sun *et al.,* 1994).

2.1.2   *Somatosensory evoked potentials (SEP)*

(1) Stimulation of body acupoints could induce SEP from the cerebral cortex. If a concentric mode of needle electrode was inserted into ST 36, and single square wave electro-stimulation supplied, SEP was recorded on the focal area of bilateral cerebral cortex in the somatic sensation area I and II (Xiao *et al.*, 1964).

(2) Applying Electro-Acupuncture (EA) on LI 4-PC 6 could induce the excitement of the central nervous fibers, of which the impulse would be conducted along specific conductive system to the contralateral cortical somatic sensation area. With the increase of the EA stimulation frequency rate, the central level became higher the longer the latent period of the induced potential, the smaller the amplitude, suggesting that high frequency EA stimulation on the cortical somatic sensation area produces inhibitive function. Increasing the intensity of EA stimulation, could expand various induced SEP amplitude without any bearing on the latent period while discontinuous increase of the stimulation intensity, slowed down the amplitude expansion (Yang *et al.*, 1978).

(3) Applying EA to the two acupoints, GV 14 and GV 26, of a rat with middle cerebral artery occlusion (MCAO) could obviously raise the SEP in various areas, and shorten various peak latent periods

(Xu *et al.*, 2001). Applying EA to acupoints LI 4 and its hind leg ST 36 of the rat with MCAO could obviously shorten its SEP latent period; an experiment in which EA and exercise therapy were concurrently applied to see the influence on its SEP latent period. It was discovered that applying EA after exercise could obviously shorten SEP latent period, but there was no such effect if the process was reversed, suggesting that whether EA and exercise therapy on SEP could produce coordinate function was related to the sequence of interference (Lin *et al.*, 2007).

(4) Other research on SEP showed that various senses, including pain, could induce SEP at the cerebral cortex, however, they have different characteristics: For example, pain stimulation on the middle segment of the small finger normally evoked one multi-phase wave complex, composed of seven components, namely P1, N1, P2, N2, P3, N3 and P4. Non-pain stimulation evoked SEP also had multi-phase wave complex, generally composed of P1, N1, P2, N2, P3 etc., 4–5 components. Comparing the two, pain evoked potentials of the corresponding components had shorter latent periods, greater amplitudes, and more complicated waveforms. The appearance of P3 after N3P4, a component which was absent in non-pain SEP, was in keeping with the pain bearer's complaint, suggesting that N3P4 and pain sense were closely related. The EA produced effects seemed to have inhibitory function on SEP in the later period, presenting as obvious drops in amplitude (He *et al.*, 1980).

(5) When acupuncture was applied to different acupoints, it could evoke motor potentials on different parts of the cerebral cortex. For example, when applied to a cat's "ST 36" acupoint, it could obviously inhibit saphenous nerve C type fibers afferent to somatosensory area I (Sm1), inducing cortical evoked potential (C-CEP, which could be considered as the index of slow pain response) including early and late periods inhibition: early inhibition came up right after EA, for a short sustaining period, and within 2 min, the amplitude value was quickly recovered; late inhibition came out gradually 4 min after applying EA, the greatest inhibitive effect was within 10–12 min, sustained for a longer time, and after 20 min, it nearly returned to pre-EA application level. When electrical stimulation was applied to the "ST 36"

acupoint, it could concurrently record apparent evoked potential in cerebral anterior lateral association area (ALA), while electrical stimulation to ALA could also have apparent inhibitive function on C-CEP. After applying 1% procaine to block ALA locally or venous injection of Naloxone, and then using EA on the "ST 36" acupoint, the delayed inhibitive function was apparently weakened but early inhibition was not affected, suggesting that EA on "ST 36" with reference to somatic cortex slowed down pain response. The early period inhibition and that of the late period could be different. The late period inhibitive function was produced through the associated cortex, through the release of the endogenous opioid (Feng *et al.*, 1989).

(6) Different frequencies (20, 40 Hz) with weak EA (1–2 V) had obvious inhibitory function on the thalamus. Applying 20 Hz strong EA (2–5V) had obvious inhibitory function on the cortical component of P14–N20, P25–N30 and P45–N60 amplitudes. Different frequencies (2, 20, 40 and 60 Hz) of strong EA (2–5 V) have apparent inhibitory effects on the pain component of P200–N300 amplitude, particularly at 20 Hz where the effect was remarkable and the after effect was strong and persistent. It became apparent that: (i) for subcortical component, the effect was obvious with low frequency EA; (ii) for cortical pain components, the effect was obvious with low frequency and strong EA; and (iii) for prohibition on the subcortical component and the pain component, there were obvious after effects (Zhang *et al.*, 2000). The influence of acupuncture on various levels of the article centers was not simply the function of excitement or inhibition, instead it is a rather complex physiological adjustment mechanism. While the central mechanism of cortical and subcortical reception to stimulation was different, hand twirling maneuvers and EA stimulation could have different influences along different receptive path, resulting in the differences in effect.

Within the Sm1 area, various receptive type of neurons could be responsive to EA and hand needling, but judging from the responsive neurons' distributions, the range of influence of EA is greater that of the hand needling. Even though neurons whose receptive scope at the acupoint area could have responded to some EA, they might show no response to manual needling. Some neurons, on the other hand, could have responded to hand needling but not to EA. Some other neurons might respond to EA and hand needling with opposite behaviors. For EA it seemed that low frequencies were better than high frequencies. More than half of those deep neurons that are responsive to EA and hand needling possess characteristics of muscle neurons. It is therefore considered that muscle receptors and other deep receptors might jointly take part in producing acupuncture responses (Yuan *et al.*, 1991).

2.1.3 *Acupuncture affects electrical activities of the cerebral cortex*

Applying EA (GV 14, GV 2 and ST 36; EA parameters: frequency 52 times/min with loose and dense waves, and intensity limited to inducing limbs with shaking) to a patient's cerebral cortex which had epilepic discharges caused by penicillin could have inhibitory effects. There could be reduction of seizures, tremors and duration of attack. It was also observed that inhibitory function of EA on the cerebral cortex could be blocked by Naloxone. If microdoses of Naloxone were injected into the abdominal cavity, cerebral ventricles or the gray matter surrounding midbrain aqueduct, and nucleus accumbens septi, the function of EA could be reversed. Injecting Noloxone directly into the cortical sensation movement area where penicillin was placed could also block the acupuncture effect, suggesting that this process involves the participation of endorphins (Wu *et al.*, 1986).

Using domestic rabbit's spontaneous electrical activities of the brain and rhythmic assimilation of electroencephalic response to repeated flashing as the index, an experiment was carried out to explore the association of acupoint (PC 6) and cerebral cortical function, and related neurological mechanisms. The results showed that EA initiated two types of response: one was the α type rhythm with high range, while the slow wave was reduced, and disappeared; while the other type initiated no obvious change. Repeated flashing usually brings out the occipitothalamic rhythm simulation response. After applying EA for one min, flashing stimulation was given concurrently. The result was intensified electroencephalographic simulation response, extending the time of rhythmic simulation with increasingly high amplitude. There was no such induced change when EA was applied to non-acupoints of the front limbs. When the plexiform nerve of the ipsilateral arm was cut off, the influence of EA on spontaneous electroencephalic and flashing light induced rhythmic simulation response could no longer appear (Zhang *et al.*, 1984).

2.1.4   *Acupoints function could be related to cerebral cortical function*

The relationship between specific group of functional acupoints and their corresponding cerebral cortex areas have been studied. EA had been applied to GB 37, TE 5 in an exploration of the relationship between the acupoints and the corresponding cerebral cortex, employing functional Magnetic Resonance Imaging (fMRI). The data obtained were analyzed by Software Project Manager (SPM) from which pictures of the brain activation was produced in terms of the contrast between messages sent under stimulating state and static conditions. The acupuncture activated areas of the cerebral cortex could thus be labeled:

(1) It was found that when EA was applied to the right lateral acupoints, GE 37 and TE 7, fMRI activities were apparently increased from his visual cortex to the inferior parietal cortex near the bilateral occipital sulcus (Qiu *et al.*, 2005).

(2) Using magnetic resonance Blood Oxygen Level Dependent (BOLD) technique as a basis to evaluate the physiological response of the cerebral cortex under the influence of acupuncture, the resulting discoveries were as follows: Among all the volunteers who received the test, it was found that all have sourness, numbness and distending symptoms. When acupuncture was applied to the left GE 37, the contralateral occipital cortex visual area appeared activated, and the contralateral basal ganglia area was also activated. When it was applied to the right lateral acupoint GB 34, the contralateral occipital cortex visual area could apparently be activated; and when it was applied to left lateral acupoint ST 36, the contralateral hypothalamus area as well as the ipsilateral hippocampus area were activated. When applied to left lateral acupoint ST 32, the ipsilateral frontal area was apparently activated (Cai *et al.*, 2007).

(3) It was evident that different acupoints along the same meridian when stimulated, might induce similar central brain effects, whereas acupoints along different meridians could have different corresponding brain areas (Fang *et al.*, 2005).

2.2 Influence of Acupuncture on Spinal Cord Function

(1) Electro activities of spinal cord. Applying EA to acupoints around the lumbar region have obvious inhibitory effects on the gastrocnemius reflex discharge while stimulating ipsilateral gastrocnemius muscle or stimulating the skin of ipsilateral lower limb. The inhibitory effects manifested as a extended latent period of discharge, a drop in the potential range or complete absence of discharge.

Regardless of where the points of stimulation were, they all had inhibitory effects on the induced somatic reflex discharge. It could therefore be considered that the range of somatic reflex initiated through acupuncture in the lumbar spine was not limited to polysynaptic reflex. It could also inhibit monosynaptic reflexes irrespective of what happened in the process of such inhibition, including pre-synaptic and post-synaptic inhibitions (Xu *et al.*, 1980).

(2) The spinal dorsal horn neuron of the cat spontaneous motion of which the discharge can be used as an index to observe the influence of applying EA to the left lateral acupoints, "ST 36" and "SP 6" affecting the left lateral greater splanchnic nerve which induces neuronic influences on stomach expansions. The results indicated that: (i) spinal chord dorsal horn neurons could receive messages and give responds stomach expansion, greater splanchnic nerve, activity, acupoints "ST 36" and "SP 6". The four kinds of messages could merge and integrate within the same spinal chord dorsal horn region; (ii) there are more neurons responding to "ST 36" than to "SP 6" during acupuncture, and some dorsal horn neurons could simultaneously accept afferent stimuli from acupoints "ST 36" and "SP 6". However, the resulting discharges were not identical, indicating that there were relative specificities related to the acupoints; (iii) it was also observed in the experiment that applying EA to acupoint "ST 36" could reverse or antagonize the changes of spinal

dorsal horn neurons induced by stomach expansion, thus leading to acupuncture analgesia; and (iv) one characteristic of acupuncture was that it produced duplex adjustment effects: excited neurons due to stomach expansion and electrical stimulation of greater splanchnic nerve on the contrary inhibit their own discharges when EA was applied to "ST 36". Those neurons inhibitory stomach expansion could revert to exciting discharge on EA stimulating of the greater splanchnic nerve when EA was applied to "ST 36" (Zhang *et al.*, 2001).

2.3 Acupuncture and Central Neurotransmitters

The regulating effects of acupuncture on the central nervous system are all related to neurotransmitter of the central nervous system. There are many varieties of central neurotransmitter, and at present those involved in the research on acupuncture included GABA, 5-hydroxytryptamine (5-HT), Dopamine (DA), nor adrenaline (NA), acetylcholinesterase (AChE), etc. In the research on EA, where $AICl_3$ poisoning of rats caused the animal's loss of learning memory, it was found that EA raised the content of Acetylcholine (Ach) and AChE in the cerebral cortex of the rat, suggesting that EA could be improving the memory disturbance through changes with the neurotransmitters (Feng *et al.*, 2003). Other experiments indicated that applying EA to MCAO rats could raise the activity of AChE in the cerebral cortex and hippocampus, while antagonizing the injury effects of the cerebral ischemia (Po *et al.*, 2002).

Studies on the mechanism of acupuncture analgesia have also found that the effects are related to many kinds of neurotransmitters, such as ACh, GABA, CCK-8, 5-HT, DA and NE, including the release of many kinds of endogenous endorphins.

2.4 Acupuncture and the Peripheral Nervous System

In the process of acupuncture therapy, the peripheral nervous system plays an integral role which includes the afferent transmissions and the feelings of "acuaesthesia". Neurotransmitters are also involved in the effective processes of acupuncture.

2.4.1 *Nerve fibers in acupuncture treatment*

Some experiments used domestic rabbit's reflex jaw movements as pain response. EA stimulations were given to ipsilateral peroneal nerve and ulnar nerve at frequencies of 45 Hz, and 2 Hz, respectively. Starting with the A α β wave group, increasing step by step until A δ wave reached the largest amplitude, and then stimulation was shifted to the C wave excitement. The acupuncture analgesia effect of various types of afferent fibers was studied. The experiment involved four observation groups, viz, proximal segment low frequency group stimulating the ulnar nerve, proximal segment high frequency group for peroneal nerve, distal segment low frequency group stimulating the ulnar nerve, and distal segment high frequency group stimulating ulnar nerve. It was found that:

(1) When applying distal low EA to all kinds of fibers, certain analgesia effects were produced: the smaller the fibers, the stronger the effects; with proximal high EA, types I and II fibers had good analgesia effect; with the addition of type III fiber stimulation analgesic effects were not strengthened. However, when EA strength was increased, exciting also the type IV fibers, the analgesic effect was apparently strengthened again. With distal low EA, types I and II fibers did not produce obvious analgesic effect, but adding excitement types III and IV fibers, there was a successive increase. With distal high EA, only exciting type IV fibers could give analgesic effect.

(2) A further observation on the changes of high low frequencies A δ amplitude, it was found that EA, at 2 Hz low frequency was not affected. The δ wave was not affected EA at 45 Hz frequency under the condition of the same strength of stimulation, showed a drop of A δ wave. The weakening of type III fibers activity at high frequency of EA, and the decrease of afferent pulsation could be the direct cause of weaker analgesic effect.

(3) In the experiments where high frequency EA excited type I, II, III and IV fibers produced good analgesic effects, after injecting Naloxone for 5 min. there was no obvious weakening of analgesic effect. Upon further waiting for 7.5 min. and 10 min, however, the analgesic effect was weakened by 57.59% and 63.49% respectively. When EA was stopped, their weaning process was accelerated, and after 5 min. it returned to the pre-EA level, indicating that Naloxone partially reversed the analgesic effect.

The following conclusions could be drawn:

(1) The EA analgesic effects of different afferent fibers under different conditions still stick to the same rule: the smaller the exciting fibers, the stronger the analgesic effect.

(2) The effects of large fibers (types I and II fibers) have obvious segmental characteristics, while the effect of small fibers (types III and IV fibers) is super segmental, working mainly through the activation of endogenous morphinoid analgesic system.

(3) High frequency EA could apparently weaken the afferent activity of small fibers, weakening or even completely negating the effects of type III fibers. The weakening on effects type IV fibers, though not too severe, yet with stress influences contributing, remains unreliable. For acupuncture analgesia and acupuncture-anaesthesia, the proximal segments, low frequency and high intensity EA should be applied to in order to achieve the most desirable analgesic effect (Tang *et al.*, 1983).

2.4.2 *Acupuncture and recovery of injured nerves*

A mouse suffering from sciatic nerve damage was used as a model to test the effect of EA therapy. The lateral GB 30 and ST 36, were stimulated with intermittent waves, at 3 Hz frequency, current intensity of 20 mA, just strong enough to, initiate slight muscle twitches. Ten min of stimulation was given once daily, six times a week, for a total of four weeks. After completion of treatment, the recovery of the sciatic nerve was found to be better than the group using the medicine and the control group. Histological observations showed that in the EA group, there was an increase of cells in the anterior horns of both L4 and L6 levels of the spinal chord and spinal ganglion. The recovery rate of the gastrocneminus muscles was also increased, as was shown in their wet weights, the diameter of the muscle cells, etc. The results suggested that EA has contributed to the functional recovery of nerve injury by promoting the regeneration of nerve cells (Shao *et al.*, 2000).

2.5 Summary and Discussion

Acupuncture theory maintained that meridians link up viscera, organs, limbs and various orifices through longitudinal channels to form an organic whole, and it is obvious that the meridian system is an important supporting view in Chinese Medicine. It might appear that the nervous system of Life Science and meridian system of Chinese Traditional Medicine (CTM) have similar characteristics, so people naturally link up meridian system with nervous system, and have conducted a great deal of research, the results of which support the relationship with nervous system at different levels. The relationship was expressed on many levels, from the cerebral cortex, different anatomical structures of the cerebrum (diencephalon, middle brain, brain stem, and cerebellum), medulla oblongata, spinal chord and peripheral afferent and efferent nerves. Nevertheless, special emphasis should be made that the meridian system of acupuncture is not entirely equivalent to the nervous system. Although many clinical effects of acupuncture could be explained with neurological principles, however, no comprehensive explanation of the clinical effects of acupuncture could be explained solely with neurological principles. In fact the therapeutic effect of acupuncture involves not only the nervous system, but also the endocrine and immunological systems. Moreover, there are many acupuncture phenomena which cannot be entirely explained with modern medical knowledge, such as getting *qi* from needling, following the meridian for effect transmission, feeling the function of needling through manual manipulation, etc. Therefore, no matter which method has been used to study the mechanisms of traditional acupuncture, one should avoid blindly equating acupuncture with simple theories of modern medicine. The characteristics of Chinese Medicine (the holistic concept and multiple targets) have paved the way to the adoption of a multilevel and crisscrossed theory, with complex associations between different levels physiological activities involving both broad neurological and humoral systems.

References

Bai, Z., Zhou, L., Zheng, H., *et al.* (2002) Influence of electroacupuncture points on AChE activity of hippocampus and cortex caused by cerebral ischemia-reperfusion rats. *J. Jinan University (Nat. Sci. Med.)* **23**(5), 101–104.

Cai, K., Chen, M., Wang, W., *et al.* (2007) fMRI of cortical activation by acupuncture. *Inform. Med. Equip.* **22**(6), 84–86.

Fang, J., Jin, Z., Wang, Y., *et al.* (2005) Comparison of central effects of acupuncturing Taichong and nearby two acupoints by functional MRI. *Chin. J. Med. Imag. Tech.* **21**(9), 1332–1336.

Feng, J. and Chen, P. (1989) Role of cerebral association area in the inhibition of electro-acu-punture on respone of somatosensory cortex to slow pain. *Acupunct. Res.* **1, 2**, 10–11.

Feng, SL., Lai, X. and Gu, J. (2003) The influence of electro-acupuncture on memory be-havior of rats acetylcholine and acetylcholin esterase in cerebral cortex. *New J. Tradit. Chin. Med.* **35**(8), 76–78.

He, G. and Xia, L. (1980) Research of evoked brain electrical caused by the human painful and non-painful stimulation. *Acupunct. Res.* **2**, 135–139.

Lin, D. and Zhang, X. (2007) Effects of different intervention order of electroacupuncture and rehabilitation training on the SEP of MCAO Rats. *J. Fujian Coll. Tradit. Chin. Med.* **17**(6), 43–45.

Po, Z., Zhou, L., Zheng, H., *et al.* (2002) Influence of electroacupuncture points on ACheE activity of hippocampus and cortex caused by cerebral ischemia–reperfusion rats. *J. Jinan Univ. (Nat. Sci. Med. Ed.)* **23**(5), 101–104.

Qiu, M., Wang, J., Xie, B., *et al.* (2005) Establishment of analyzing methods for functional MR images when electroacupuncture stimulation on Guangming and Waiguan acu-points. *Acta Academiae Medicinae Militaris Tertiae* **27**(19), 1970–1972.

Shao, S., Shan, B., Yan, Z., *et al.* (2000) Experimental study on electro-acupuncture ther-apy promoting the regeneration of the rats injured sciatic nerve. *Mod. Rehabil.* **4**(8), 1184–1185.

Sun, Z., Huo, L., Liu, L., *et al.* (1994) Study on meproduced by acupucture scalp. *Chin. J. Tradit. Med. Sci. Tech.* **1**(6), 14–19.

Tang, J., Hu, A. and Hou, Z. (1983) The role and its mechanism of the Electroacupuncture through various types of afferent fibers under different conditions. *J. Xi'an Jiaotong Univ. (Med. Sci.)* **4**(1), 1–7.

Wu, D., Ma, J. and Li, W. (1976) Inhibitory effect of electroacupuncture on the cerebral cortex epileptiform discharges induced by penicillin. *Acta Physiologica Sinica* **38**(3), 325–331.

Xiao, J., Luo, F., *et al.* (1964) Research of stimulation of rabbit "Zusanli" site and the evoked potentials of the cerebral cortex. *J. Peking Univ. (Health Sci.)* **1**, 6–10.

Xu, M., Zhang, L. and Xu, T. (1980) Analysis of the interspinous point inhibiting the spinal reflex discharge. *J. Harbin Med. Univ.* **2**, 10–12.

Xu, N., Shen, D., Zhou, Y., *et al.* (2001) Effects of electroacupuncture on cortical somato-sensory evoked potential and cellular ultrastructure in rats of local cerebral ischemia. *J. Tradit. Chin. Med.* **42**(6), 342–344, 354.

Yang, S., Ma, Z., Dong, C., *et al.* (1980) Electro-acupuncture stimulation and evoked potentials of somatosensory. *J. Hebei Med. Univ.* **1**(1), 11–16.

Yuan, B., Pang, T. and Liu, X. (1991) Response properties of SI cortical neurons to electro-acupuncture and manual acupuncture in the rat. *Acupunct. Res.* **2**, 79–85.

Zhang, J., Jin, Z., Lu, B. *et al.* (2001) Responses of spinal dorsal-horn neurons to gastric disten-tion and electroacupuncture of "Zusanli" point. *Acupunct. Res.* **26**(4), 268–271.

Zhang, L., Cheng, J. and Yan, J. (2000) Observation on the characteristics of different central somatosensory evoked potentials after the stimulation by electro-acupuncture. *J. Beijing Univ. Tradit. Chin. Med.* **23**(6), 43–45.

Zhang, S., Qu, J., Zhang, M. (1984) The impact of electro-acupuncture points on the EEG of rabbits. *Basic Med. Sci. Clin.* **4**(5,6), 91.

Chapter 3

Acupuncture for Immunomodulation

Abstract

The human immunological system provides important endogenous mechanisms of defense against invading organisms and unbalanced physiological activities. One of the important immunological functions is concerned with the clearing of foreign proteins (antigens). When the organism is stimulated by an antigen coming from outside, its immunological system reacts by producing an antibody against the antigen with the aim of getting rid of it. Foreign antigens include non-pathogenic antigens (such as pollen), invasive microorganism and the toxins it produces, and degraded cell products produced by the organism itself, including those cells undergoing cancerous changes. The physiological balance being enjoyed by the living organism depends on the effective function of its immunological system. Immunological activities function in three ways: viz. immuno-defense, immuno-monitoring, and immuno stabilization. These activities take place within the cells or outside.

Acupuncture affects immunological function in two directions: either strengthening the weak responses; or in case of over-excessive responses regulating or inhibiting the over activities.

Keywords: Immunomodulation; Physiological Balance; Immunological Functions.

3.1 Acupuncture and Cellular Immune Function

3.1.1 *Acupuncture activates T cells and related sub-groups*

(1) When Electro-Acupuncture (EA) was given to normal volunteers' ST 36, GB 34 or ST 36 and ST 40, there was an increase of T lymphocytes in the peripheral blood, and strengthened esterase activations in the T lymphocytes. The observation was the same for both young and old

people (Huang *et al.*, 1984). Similarly, stimulating two groups of acupoints ST 15, ST 36 and CV 16; or SI 11, GB 21 and BL 23, led to strengthening of the T lymphocytes of patient with mazoplasia, and at the same time promoting the transformation of normal lymphocyte into lymphoblast (Ma *et al.*, 1980).

(2) EA given principally to EX-B2 and supported by standard puncturing for bronchial asthma patient for four weeks led to an increase of the total number of T lymphocytes (CD_3^+) and T helper cells (CD_4^+) with obvious improvement of CD_4^+/CD_8^+ ratio (Han 2000).

(3) Using moxibustion on GV 14, BL 13 and BL 20 of a cancer patient, it was observed that the lymphocytes transformation rate was increased without affecting the absolute value of CD_3^+, CD_4^+ and CD_8^+, while the ratio of CD_4^+/CD_8^+, was increased (Zhai, 1994).

(4) When EA was applied to ST 36 of a rat under immuno-inhibition of its pituitary gland, the rats suppressed ir-SP content and CD_4^+ in its peripheral blood resumed to normal. When a normal rat was similarly treated with EA on ST 36, ir-SP and CD_4^+ were raised (Gao *et al.*, 2001).

Acupuncture and moxibustion on T cells could have strengthened the activation of T lymphocytes, promoted the activation of esterase in T lymphocytes, and promoted the transformation of normal lymphocytes. In addition the T cell subgroups showed increases in CD_3^+ and CD_4^+, and CD_4^+/CD_8^+ ratio without apparent changes in CD_8^+.

3.1.2 *Acupuncture activates NK cells*

(1) Direct moxibustion on acupoints, GV 14, BL 13 and BL 20, of a cancer patient showed that his natural killer cells (NK cells), which had low activity, were strengthened (Zhai *et al.*, 1994).

(2) Marathon runners were found to have a decrease in the number of NK cells after four hours running extending to 28 hours. When EA was given at CV 4, ST 36, and SP 6, four hours after the competition, using a continuous wave, frequency at 80–100/s. for 30 min, a small increase in NK cells was found in the blood of the runner 28 hours after. It was suggested that the immune system after a temporary inhibition during a vigorous race, was helped by acupuncture for a quick recovery (Zhu *et al.*, 2007).

(3) Experiments on mice under artificial stress conditions revealed suppressed NK cell activities in their spleen and thymus, and IL-2 activity was lower than normal. EA given to the thymus of the mice around "CV 17", "CV 18", "CV 19", "CV 20", "CV 21" and "CV 22", was able to raise the activity of both NK cells and IL-2 (Yuan *et al.*, 2002).

(4) Experiments on animals found that acupuncture on ST 36, CV 17, GV 14; and CV 4, ST 15 could strengthen the NK cell activities of a mouse after transplantation of breast cancer cells. At the same time, its T lymphocytes, acid α-naphthyl acetate esterase (α-ANAE) level, lymphocyte transformation rate, and infiltration of lymphocytes were all raised (Liu *et al.*, 1995).

3.1.3 *Acupuncture and macrophages*

(1) When EA was applied to bilateral ST 36 and CV 4 of a rat, the index of macrophage in the liver of the rat was raised. EA on an old rat tended to increase the number of macrophages so that when compared with the young rat, little change was obvious. Acupuncture not only increased the number of macrophages in the liver of an old rat, but also converted them to the activated state (Zhu *et al.*, 2003).

(2) Immuno-deficient models of mice were created with cytotoxic drug administration or artificial virus infection. When such model was treated for three days on GV 14 with EA, the death rate was lowered and the survival was extended. Examination showed raised serum interferon and raised phagocytic macrophages (Chou *et al.*, 1990).

The regulating functions of acupuncture and moxibustion on macrophage are reflected in the following aspects: increase in quantity, enlargement of volume, strengthening of phagocytic ability, and converting them to an activated state.

3.1.4 *Acupuncture and leukocyte phagocytosis*

(1) 142 patients suffering from bacillary dysentery were divided into an acupuncture and moxibustion group (115 cases treated on acupoints, ST 25, CV 10, CV 4, CV 8 by moxibustion, ST 36, and CV 6), and a medicine control group (27 cases treated with furazolidone). After

treatment for nine days, the acupuncture and moxibustion group attained an average curing rate of 83.47% and average curing time of 4.47 days; apparently the result was better than that of the medicine group. From the laboratory test, it was found that after acupuncture and moxibustion, the bactericidal ability of the plasma was raised. Three days after acupuncture-moxibustion treatment, the low phago-cytic activity of white cells were raised to a higher level than normal, and was also better compared with the medicine group (TCM Acupuncture-Moxibustion Research Institute, Gansu Province TCM Hospital, 1985).

(2) When EA (current strength at 2 mA, frequency 187 Hz, for 15 min) was applied to a healthy horse's acupoint, GV 20, etc., after 24 hours, it was found that the phagocytic ability of the white cells was obvi-ously strengthened. When the horse was subjected to blister beetles bites to produce local inflammation, EA treatment improved the white cell phagocytic ability in the venous blood. The experiment suggested that there was a multiplicity of impact of acupuncture on the phago-cytic ability of white cells, related to the organism's general condi-tions. Acupuncture also helped to smoothen the horse's inflammatory reactions (The Experimental Research Group on Anti-inflammation, Shen Hou Army Horse Diseases Prevention Research Institute, 1982).

There might be a duplex regulatory effect of acupuncture and moxibustion on the phagocytosis of white cells: to those white cells whose phagocytosis was weak, acupuncture gives strengthening; to those white cells whose phagocytosis is over-excited, acupuncture gives inhibition, thus relieving the living organism from over-reaction to inflammation.

3.1.5 *Acupuncture and red blood cells*

The immune function of red cells is primarily achieved through the cir-culating immune complex (CIC) of the C3b receptor on the membrane adhesive in the blood circulation, moving it to liver and spleen, promot-ing phagocytes to eliminate CIC, and preventing the deposit of CIC in the tissues of the organism and causing disease. There were experiments in which it was found that the chance for CIC in the blood circulation to encounter red cells is 500–1000 times more than the white cells. This leads to the assumption that the red cells immune adherence function mainly depends on RBC-C3bRR and RBC-ICR (Guo *et al.*, 1982). In one experiment, acupuncture was applied to the rabbit. After three days, it was found that the rabbit's RBC-C3bRR and RBC-ICR were both raised, the effect sustained for more than 24 hours.

When EA was applied to ST 36 of an immunosuppressed rat, the RBC-C3bRR and RBC-ICR of the animal were raised. The application of EA to ST 36 of a normal rat could also raise the positive regulating function of the peripheral T lymphocytes and the immune adherence ability of the red cells (Gao *et al.*, 2000).

3.2 Acupuncture and Humoral Immune Function

3.2.1 *Acupuncture regulates specific immunoglobulin*

Immunoglobulin is the protein basis of humoral immunity. Complement is a specific humoral immunity factor, and it has the important function of expanding specific immune responses. The occurrence and development of rheumatoid arthritis (RA) is related to the auto-immunity process.

(1) Acupuncture and moxibustion therapies, mainly on CV 4, CV 6, ST 36, BL 18, BL 23, and BL20 could improve such symptoms as joint pain, motion pain, swelling and stiffness, etc. Acupuncture reduces the levels of IgA, IgG and IgM in blood serum, while moxibustion can be superior to simple acupuncture therapy, as evidenced from clinical therapy (86.21% vs. 57.14%) (Liu *et al.*, 2006). Asthma patients' IgG in serum were found to be lower than normal levels while IgM and IgE were higher than normal. After treating with acupuncture and moxibustion for one month, IgG was increased, and IgM and IgE were reduced (Zhang *et al.*, 1993).

(2) Using acupuncture and moxibustion together with hot cupping as combined treatment, patients with allergic asthma responded with better control of SIgA and lower IgA in the saliva and nose secretions. After acupuncture and moxibustion therapy, IgE levels in patients' serum were obviously lowered than that before treatment, a drop of 54%, suggested that patients suffering from allergic asthma due to

mast cell over-reaction producing IgE could be controlled with acupuncture (Yang *et al.*, 1995).

(3) When acupoint ST 36 was injected with anti-allergic fluid, not only was the clinical therapeutic effect apparently higher than that of the anti-allergic agent, but the patient's serum total IgE was also reduced (Chen *et al.*, 1996).

The regulating effect of acupuncture and moxibustion on immunoglobulin is apparently bidirectional, irrespective of immunoglobulin's rise or fall.

3.3 Acupuncture and Tumour Immunology

Sixty-eight cases of Stage 3 cervix cancer patients receiving regular radiation therapy were randomly divided into moxibustion treatment group (radiation therapy + moxibustion, 38 cases) and control group (30 cases with radiation therapy). Acupoints chosen were: ST 36, CV 8, and SP 6 (Yu *et al.*, 2003). The results were as showed:

(1) After moxibustion, there was an increase in all IL-2, IL-6, and IL-8, of which IL-2 was most remarkable. IL-2 could induce antigen stimulated T cell proliferation and enhance the cytotoxic effects of major histocompatibility complex (MHC), and induce MHC non-restrictive lymphokine activated killer (LAK) activity of large granular lymphocytes, strengthening the tumour killing activity of NK cells, LAK cells and lymphocytes (Wu, 1996).

(2) Acupuncture and moxibustion could elevate the patient's peripheral blood $CD3^+$ and $CD4^+$ remarkably, while $CD8^+$ did not have apparent change. There was an increase in the $CD4^+/CD8^+$ ratio. T cell immunology had leading effects, through activated $CD4^+$ cells secretory factors which assist $CD8^+$ T cells in killing cancer cells (Huang *et al.*, 2000), and $CD4^+$ T cells also had direct killing effects on tumor cells (Bell *et al.*, 1998). It was evident that the inter synergism among the T cells subgroups played an important immunological role.

(3) Immunoglobulin originated from B lymphocytes take part in fluid immunity. After radiation therapy, blood IgG, IgA and IgM levels dropped in various degrees. After moxibustion therapy, IgG and IgM levels became higher. This could be related to moxibustion which

raised the number of T cells and the activity of IL-2, leading to the participation of the activation, proliferation, and differentiation of other cells, and promoting B cells to transform into effector plasma cells.

(4) RBC-C3b is the central link of the red cell immunology. Apart from recognizing antigens, it could adhere to antigens, antibodies and complements, carrying them to the liver and spleen to be eliminated.

3.4 Acupuncture and Non-specific Immunity

3.4.1 *Effect of acupuncture on complement*

(1) When EA was applied to a normal person's ST 36 and GB 34 or ST 40, it could increase the content of C4 and properdin B factor, and the effect was more remarkable in the youth than in the aged. There was no apparent change in C3 (Huang *et al.*, 1986).

(2) Ninety-two patients suffering from chronic nettle rash were divided into two groups; one group was treated with acupuncture together with medication (50 cases) and the other with medication alone (42 cases). Cetirizine 10 mg was given once daily, with or without acupuncture. Acupoints LI 4, SP 10, SP 36, and SP 6 were used for treatment which lasted for one month. The effective rate of the acupuncture plus medicine group was higher than that of the control group (73.6%). In the laboratory test, it was found that a patient suffering from chronic nettle rash had average serum complement C3 level lower than that of a healthy person. In the acupuncture and medicine group, the complement C3 level was apparently increased. There was no apparent change in the medicine group (Ai *et al.*, 2003).

The regulating function of acupuncture and moxibustion on serum complement also had a bidirectional nature, maximizing it to restore to normal.

3.5 Summary and Discussion

The regulating effects of acupuncture and moxibustion on the function of human immunological system are very extensive, and in accordance with different patients' conditions, there are important regulating effects on the network of immunological functions, including the cellular or fluid category, and such functional influences could be bidirectional.

(1) For those who are deficient in immunological activity, acupuncture and moxibustion could strengthen it. The manifestations include: (i) strengthening the activity of lymphocytes, promoting normal lymphocytes' transformation into lymphoblast; (ii) increasing the percentage between CD3 and CD4, especially raising the ratio of CD4/CD8; (iii) increasing the immunological activity of substance P; (iv) strengthening IL-2 activity, increasing the number of NK cells and strengthening their activity, activating macrophages, increasing their quantity and strengthening phagocytosis; (v) raising the valence of interferon, increasing the phagocytosis of white cells and neutrophilic cells; (vi) enhancing the immunological function of red cells by intensifying the adherent activity of red cells and C3b receptors, increasing the content of CIC and lowering the rosette inhibitive rate of red cells; (vii) raising IgG levels in an asthma patient's serum and increasing IgG and IgM levels in a tumor patient; (viii) enhancing C4 in healthy persons' serum and content of properdin B factor, and elevating the level of C3 in allergic patient's serum; and (ix) increasing the content of Lysozyme (LSZ) in serum.

(2) When immunological functions are overactive, which causes the excessive responses such as allergy, auto-immunity, hyper reactions, etc., acupuncture and moxibustion could have inhibitory effects. Examples include: (i) lowering the levels of IgA, IgG and IgM in the serum of rheumatologic patients, and reducing the levels of IgM and IgE in asthma patients; (ii) suppressing phagocytosis of white cells, reducing inflammation reactions; (iii) lowering allergic asthma patients' salivary contents of SIgA and total IgA in nose secretions, and reducing the level of IgE in serum; and (iv) lowering the serum levels of C3 and C4 in people prone to diseases. Moreover, acupuncture and moxibustion also regulates agglutinins, indirect hemoglobin agglutinin, precipitin and hemolysin, etc.

Since the human immunological system is regulated by other physiological activities, it displays different changes in the onset of diseases and during their development. When acupuncture and moxibustion are used to regulate the human immunological function, what is happening in the neurological, circulatory and endocrine systems will also be affected. At present, the research on the mechanism of actions of acupuncture and moxibustion in such activities remains rather scanty and is yet lacking systematic organization. Prescriptions on the selection of acupoints for special immunological needs are still under trial. Likewise, results of acupuncture are not guaranteed.

References

Ai, Z., Zhang, Q., Zou, T., *et al.* (2003) Effect of acupuncture on serum complement C_3 content in the patient of chronic urticaria. *Chin. Acupunct. Moxibustion* **23**(11), 641–643.

Bell, E.B., Sparshott, S.M. and Bunce, C. (1998) CD4+ T-cell memory, CD45R subsets and the persistence of antigen — a unifying concept. *Immunol. Today* **19**(2), 60–64.

Chen, L., Li, A., Tao, J., *et al.* (1996) Clinical and experimental studies on preventing and treating anaphylactic asthma with zusanli point immunotherapy. *Chin. J. Integr. Tradit. West. Med.* **16**(12), 709–712.

Chou, Y., Cao, Y., Wang, J., *et al.* (1990) Protective effect of acupuncture on influenza virus infectious mice. *China J. Tradit. Chin. Med. Pharm.* **5**(2), 16–18.

Gao, W, Huang, Y., Zhao, N., *et al.* (2000) Influences of electroacupuncture (EA) on T lymphocyte subgroups of peripheral blood and erythrocyte immune function in rats. *J. Fourth Mil. Med. Univ.* **21**(4), 414–416.

Gao, W., Huang, Y., Chen, H., *et al.* (2001) Effects of rats' ir-SP and cellular immune function while electro-puncturing rats' Zusanli points. *J. Fourth Mil. Med. Univ.* **22**(9), 793–796.

Guo, F., Li, C., Zhao, Z., *et al.* (1982) Preliminary study on immune function of normal human red cells. *Acad. J. Second Mil. Med. Univ.* **3**, 188–190.

Han, A. (2000) The impact of acupuncture on cellular immune function in patients with bronchial asthma. *J. Clin. Acupunct. Moxibustion* **16**(4), 53–54.

Huang, H., Yu, H. and Lin, Y. (2000) Anti-tumor effect of CD4+ T cells. *Foreign Med. Sci.* **23**(1), 51–53.

Huang, K., Rong, X., Cai, H., *et al.* (1986) Observation of the effects of electroacupuncture (EA) on Some components of complement system in normal man. *Acupuncture Res.* **4**, 294–229.

Huang, K.H., Rong, X.D. and Cai, H. (1984) The observation of electro-acupuncture on human peripheral blood T lymphocytes. *Acupuncture Res.* **4**, 290–293.

Liu, J. and Ju, Y. (2006) Clinical observation of temperature acupuncture treatment of rheumatoid arthritis. *Shanghai J. Acupunct. Moxibustion* **25**(7), 23–24.

Liu, L., Guo, C., Jiao, X., *et al.* (1995) Effect of acupuncture on immunologic function and histopathology of transplanted mammary cancer in mice. *Chin. J. Integr. Tradit. West. Med.* **15**(10), 615–617.

Ma, Z., Chong, H. and Yao, Z. (1980) Experimental observation of effects of acupuncture on cellular immune function. *Shaanxi Med. J.* **9**(7), 56–59.

TCM (1985) Acupuncture-moxibustion research institute, Gansu province traditional chinese medicine hospital. Clinical observation and mechanism study of acupuncture treatment for acute bacillary dysentery. *J. Med. Res.* **14**(6), 181–182.

The Experimental Research Group on Anti-inflammation, Shen Hou Army Horse Diseases Prevention Research Institute. (1982) Observation of electro-acupuncture on leukocyte phagocytic function of horses and mules. *Chin. J. Vet. Sci. Tech.* **3**, 22–23.

Wu, J. and Huang, D. (1996) Research overview of acupuncture in regulating IL-2-IFN-OF NKC immune network. *Chin. Acupunct. Moxibustion*, **16**(6), 54–56.

Yang, Y., Chen, H., Zhao, C., *et al.* (1995) Studies on regulatory effects of acupuncture on mucosal secretory IgA in patients with Allergic Asthma. *Acupuncture Res.* **20**(2), 68–70.

Yu, Z., Wang, H. and Xu, L. (2003) Effect of moxibustion on immunologic function in patients with cervical carcinoma in radiotherapy. *Modern J. Integr. Tradit. Chin. West. Med.* **12**(24), 2629–2630.

Yuan, H., Yuan, L. and Ma, H. (2002) Effect of acupuncture on the cellular immune function of the rat under stress state. *Acupuncture Res.* **27**(3), 211–213.

Zhai, D., Chen, H. and Wang, R. (1994) Observation of direct moxibustion in regulation of cellular immune function of cancer patients. *J. Clin. Acupunct. Moxibustion*, **10**(01), 25–27.

Zhang, J., Guan, Z. and Guan, Z. (1993) The experimental study of acupuncture adjusting the humoral immune function. *Chin. Med. Materia Medica*, **14**(5), 22–25.

Zhu, M., Gao, H. and Liu, R. (2003) The experimental research on the Kupffer cell function in liver by acupuncturing "Zusanli"and "Guanyuan"of old rats. *J. Clin. Acupunct. Moxibustion*, **9**(6), 52–54.

Zhu, Z. and Chen, P. (2007) Four hours after the half-marathon, the variation of immune cells when interfering with acupuncture. *J. Shanghai Univ. Sport* **31**(2), 64–66.

Chapter 4

Acupuncture for Endocrine Function

Abstract

The effect of acupuncture on the human endocrine function could have many ways of manifestation, including direct promotion of hormonal release or through the hypothalamic-pituitary-endocrine axis. This might reflects the "holistic concept" of the fundamental theory of Chinese Medicine. Diseases may be caused directly by disorders of the human endocrine system when insufficient or excessive secretions of hormones occur. Diseases may also initiate a relative excess or insufficient endocrine secretion. The adjustment effects of acupuncture on the endocrine function could be an initiation of enhancement or inhibition.

Keywords: Endocrine; Hormones.

4.1 Regulating Effects of Acupuncture on the Endocrine System

The endocrine system is made up of a number of endocrine glands, the secretions of which produce general effects on all organs. The active substance secreted by the endocrine glands and related tissues is called hormone. Hormones are directly released into blood and tissue fluid by glandular cells of the endocrine system, after which they circulate to different parts of the whole body. Hormonal influence covers the activities of all physiological areas including general metabolism, function of tissue and organ, growth and development, reproduction, aging, etc. The normal physiological function of other systems like gastrointestinal, hematological, renal, neurological and cardiac are all under hormonal control. The common hormones include thyrotropin-releasing hormone (TRH), corticotropin-releasing hormone (CRH), gonadotropin-releasing hormone (GnRH), and growth hormone releasing hormone (GHRH), released by hypothalamus; adrenocorticotropic hormone (ACTH), growth hormone (GH), Prolactin (PRL), thyroid stimulating hormone (TSH), follicle stimulating hormone (FSH) and luteinizing hormone (LH) by adenohypophysis, thyroxine (T4) and T3 by thyroid, sex hormone, adrenaline and arterenol by adrenal and insulin (INS) by islet, etc. Excessive or deficient production of any hormone, will immediately lead to specific pathological condition (Sun *et al.*, 2003).

A great deal of clinical and experimental results have been published which show that attempts have been made on the use of acupuncture for the treatment of different hormonal pathology.

4.2 Regulating Effects of Acupuncture on the Hypothalamic-Pituitary-Adrenals (HPA) Endocrine Axis

"Preventive moxibustion" (逆灸) is one of the "sickness prevention" methods advocated since ancient China, referring to the application of moxibustion in advance when the organism is still healthy, before the outbreak of pathology. The traditional method was used to stimulate the *qi* of meridians to strengthen the human body to cope with changes, maintain health and prevent falling sick.

(1) Using the method of forced swimming in cold water, rats were initiated to fall into a state of chronic fatigue syndrome (CFS). The function of the HPA axis of these rats was studied through the secretion of CRH and acupuncture was used to influence the CFS. Acupoints chosen were GV 20 and ST 36, and Electro-Acupuncture (EA) was used with 6 V voltage, producing dispersed and dense waves of 2/20 Hz frequency, while the intensity was limited to slight vibration of the local skin and muscles. It was observed the rats developed raised hypothalamus, pituitary, and adrenal gland indices after acupuncture. Molecular expression of CRH, pituitary CRH, and mRNA were elevated. After EA therapy, the index of adrenal gland dropped, but there was no apparent change in the hypothalamus and pituitary indices, although the levels of hypothalamic CRH and mRNA and the content of CRH were lowered. (Chen *et al.*, 2007).

(2) In a study to explore the mechanism of EA on anti-depression, 100 patients with depression were randomly divided into an EA treatment group and a medicine treatment group. For the EA group, the following acupoints were selected: GB 12 and LR 3, with the following EA parameters: high frequency, dispersed and dense wave, intensity was used within the patient's endurance limit, while during the acupuncture, the frequency was increased many times to maintain the continuity of EA stimulating sensation. For the medicine group, Sertraline 50 mg was given. Both groups were treated for 12 weeks. Assessments were given before and on 2nd, 4th, and 12th weeks. Serum ACTH plasma and cortisol (COR) were detected before and after treatment. The results indicated that both treatment methods lowered depression score, and the plasma ACTH and COR were gradually lowered to normal. There was no apparent difference between the two groups (Wang *et al.*, 2007).

(3) There was one study on obesity, where EA was applied to 61 obese patients. Their fasting blood sugar (FBS), triglyceride (TG) and total cholesterol (TC) were higher than normal people while their blood cortisol (BCS), salivary cortisol (SCS) and blood adrenaline (Ad) were apparently lower than normal people. After EA, there was better weight loss. At the same time, there was elevation of BCS, SCS and Ad, while BS, TG and TC dropped, suggesting that the acupuncture could have modulated the mechanism of HPA axis in patients of simple obesity (Liu *et al.*, 1991).

4.3 Regulating Effects of Acupuncture on the Hypothalamic-Pituitary-Gonadal (HPG) Endocrine Axis

The neuroendocrine regulation of menstrual cycles is a very complicated process. The function of the hypothalamic-pituitary-ovary axis not only has direct control but also entertains the reverse influences. Positive and negative feedback help to maintain the promotion and restraint to maintain the normal gonadal function. In the normal menstrual cycle, prior to ovulation the content of serum FSH and LH is maintained at a low level. During the follicular stage, the follicles in the ovary gradually mature and produce estradiol (E2), which reaches the first physiological peak before ovulation.

At the progestational stage, the second lower peak is formed. Both peaks rise rapidly, but after ovulation they both rapidly return to the original level at the follicular stage. Progesterone (P) and estriol (E3) are responsible for endometrial changes between proliferative stage and progestational stage. At the same time, they conversely affect the hypothalamus and pituitary, regulating their secretion of FSH and LH.

Male hormone is also a very important hormone in the female reproductive physiology and functions as a precursor of female hormone. However, when there is too much male hormone in the female body, it could be harmful, disturbing the normal menstrual activities and possibly also causing obesity and disturbances in sugar and fat metabolism.

(1) A study was conducted to investigate the influence of EA on the reproductive endocrine function of a healthy female. EA treatment was applied to 28 cases of healthy females to find out the changes in the levels of FSH, LH, E_2, testosterone (T) and P, etc. The treatment started three days before the expected ovulation day, and was given once daily, lasting four days. The acupoints selected included CV 5, SP 6, ear acupoints G4. The results indicated that after acupuncture, there was no apparent change in FSH and LH, but E_2, T and P all apparently dropped, suggesting that acupuncture has no apparent influence on the secretion of gonadotropin from the pituitary in healthy females, while there was an apparent inhibitory effect on the secretion of ovarian hormones (Li *et al.*, 2003).

(2) There are abnormal changes of endocrine function in patients suffering from malignant tumors. After radiochemotherapy, the disturbance of endocrine function is further aggravated. A clinical study on 114 cases of radiochemotherapy showed that the endocrine changes included a decline of COR, increase in E2 and E3, and increase in T among female patients. EA was mainly done on acupoints: LI 11, LI 4, ST 36 and SP 6. Treatment lasted 20 days, one treatment daily (Yang *et al.*, 1995).

(3) It was found in an animal study that one week prior to ovulation, when acupuncture was applied to a female rhesus monkey, once daily, seven days in a row, there was a definite inhibitory effect on the level of pituitary gonadotropin (i.e. LSH and LH), E2 and T in the peripheral blood (Li *et al.*, 1999).

Other experiments on oophorectomized rats using acupoints CV 4, CV 3, SP 6 and EX-CA 1 was conducted using EA. Continuous wave, at frequency at 2–3 Hz, 1–2 mA, was used, to produce slight vibration of the animal's lower limbs. The following observations were observed: (i) There was an increase in the argentaffin granules, AgNORs in the organizing zone of the chromo some centre of the adrenal cortex of the rats, and an increase in the level of blood adrenal gland steroid hormones (Chen *et al.*, 1994). (ii) EA could increase the levels of E_2 and pituitary ER and mRNA in the rat (Li *et al.*, 1998). (iii) After the removal of the ovary for 3–4 weeks, there was a slight increase of enzyme activity of aromatase, an estrogen precursor in the rats fatty tissues, liver tissues and brain tissues. After applying EA, the activity of aromatase in the fat and liver tissues was further raised, the level of female E2 was obviously higher than that before the acupuncture, and the increase of brain aromatase activity was not obvious. There were no such changes in normal rats treated with EA (Cheng *et al.*, 2001). (iv) When the rat was being treated with EA, its excessive secretion of LH was apparently inhibited. It was also found after oophorectomy, the expression of its Nociceptin/Orphanin FQ (OFQ) and receptor were lowered. There was a significant increase of nociceptive immuno-positive neurons in the basal medial preoptic of the hypothalamus area and in eminence nociceptive immuno-positive tissues of the median, with an accompanying upward expression of nociceptin mRNA of the basal hypothalamus (An *et al.*, 2005).

(4) Other studies explored the relationship between EA and specific responses in the reproductive hormones, the best timing for treatment and the most effective way of application. The rats were divided into pseudo EA group, CV 4 puncture group and PC 6 puncture group. The rats were in different stages of the estrous cycle, namely estrous antephase, estrous phase and estrous anaphase respectively. Blood was collected from the rats 30 min before, during and 30 min after EA to assess the concentration of GnRH and LH. Two brain injury groups (injury and pseudo-injury to the median eminence) were also included to observe when EA was applied to "CV 4" how it would affect the regulating pattern of GnRH, LH and E2. The results indicated: (i) In the pseudo EA group, the effects of EA on the levels of GnRH and LH in the

different phases in the estrous cycle were not the same. The level of GnRH was the highest during the estrous cycle, while the level of LH was the highest in the antephase and the change of GnRH and LH were synchronized. (ii) EA increased the level of GnRH and LH in the peripheral blood, and the result was significant in the CV 4 group, and the change was more significant during the estrous phase. (iii) The regulating effect of EA on GnRH and LH appeared to be time-related, of which 30 min produced more significant effects than 60 min. (iv) After injuring the median eminence, EA could still affect GnRH level, but the regulating effect on LH and E2 levels basically disappeared (Wang *et al.*, 2007).

(5) A comparison has been made between menopausal and young animals. It was found that in the former group, E_2 level was lowered and FSH and LH were increased. When EA was applied to the menopausal animals, the serum FSH and LH levels declined and E_2 level went up. With regard to the ovarian weight, there was no significant change. It was postulated EA raised E_2 level through an increase in the secretion of adrenogenic female hormone rather than the improvement of ovarian endocrine function itself. Female hormone appeared to have a negative feedback effect on the secretion and synthesis of pituitary gonadotropin. By raising the E_2 level, EA rebuilt the negative feedback relationship between ovary and pituitary, lowering the level of gonadotropin in the blood (Liu *et al.*, 2002).

4.4 Regulating Effects of Acupuncture on the Thyroid-Pituitary Axis

Forty-six patients suffering from hyperthyrotoxicosis were treated with acupuncture. Acupoints selected included LI 18, PC 6, PC 5 and SP 36. Treatment was given once every other day, totaling 50 times as a treatment course. The study results found that 47.83% of the cases enjoyed a complete control of the symptom while the total effective rate reached 73.91%. Patients who suffered from hyperthyrotoxicosis had low serum TSH level, while T4 and T3 were significantly higher than normal. After a course of acupuncture therapy, it could seen that the serum TSH was significantly increased while T4, T3 and rT3 all significantly declined, and the decline of T4 and T3 was most remarkable.

4.5 Summary and Discussion

The effect of acupuncture on the human endocrine function could have many ways of manifestation, including direct promotion of hormonal release or through the hypothalamic-pituitary-endocrine axis. This might reflects the "holistic concept" of the fundamental theory of Chinese Medicine.

Diseases caused by disorders of the human endocrine system may be related to the insufficient or excessive secretions of hormones. The adjustment effects of acupuncture on the endocrine function could be affected through enhancement or inhibition.

Since the endocrine system has the role of regulating the functions of different organs, it follows that the use of acupuncture would tend to affect multiple pathologies. The use of acupuncture to achieve are specific endocrine disorder will be quite exceptional.

References

An, X., Ma, S., Feng, Y., *et al.* (2005) Hypothalamic orphanin FQ participated in the regulation of electroacupuncture on LH release in ovariectomized rats. *Acupunct. Res.* **30**(3), 138–142.

Chen, B., Ji, S. and Gao, H. (1994) Electro-acupuncture adjustment of hypothalamic-pituitary-ovarian axis abnormal function in ovariectomized rats. *J. Fudan Univ. (Med. Sci.)* **21**(S), 67–72.

Chen, Y., Yang, W., Fu, S., *et al.* (2007) Experimental study on expression of HPA-index and CRHmRNA with electro-acupuncture on CFS Model Rats. *Shanghai J. Acupunct. Moxibustion* **26**(2), 35–38.

Cheng, L., Du, G. and Chen, B. (2001) The Biochemical mechanism of electroacupuncture regulation of dysfunctional hypothalamic-pituitary-ovarian axis in ovariectomized rats. *Shanghai J. Acupunct. Moxibustion* **20**(6), 32–34.

Li, Y., Yang, R., Gao, H., *et al.* (1998) Influence of acupuncture on the expression of pituitary estrogen receptor mRNA and the level of blood estradiol (E-2) in the female rats. *Acupunct. Res.* **1**, 28–32.

Li, B., Huang, Y., Wang, X., *et al.* (1999) Experimental study on inhibitory effect of acupuncture on genital endocrines in the rhesus. *Chin. Acupunct. Moxibustion* **19**(8), 486–489.

Li, B., Wu, L., Xu, W., *et al.* (2003) Effects of acupuncture on reproductive endocrine system in healthy women. *Chin. Acupunct. Moxibustion* **23**(5), 293–294.

Liu, H., Wu, G., Wang, B., *et al.* (2002) Experimental research on climacteric syndrome treated by acupuncture. *J. Tianjin Coll. Tradit. Chin. Med.* **21**(1), 45–46.

Liu, Z., Xiao, S., Hu, L., *et al.* (1991) The impact of acupuncture on simple obesity adrenal. *Shanghai. J. Acupunct. Moxibustion* **3**, 7–9.

Sun, Y., Duan, W., Li, D., *et al.* (2003) *Practical Endocrine and Metabolic Diseases.* Therapeutics People's Medical Publishing House, Beijing, pp. 1–3.

Wang, S. and Zhu, B. (2007) Regulative effect of electroacupuncture on hypothalamus-hypophysis-gonad axis in different stages of estrous cycles in rats. *Acupunct. Res.* **32**(2), 119–124.

Wang, X., li·tielike, A. and Zhao, Z. (2007) The regulation of plasma adrenocorticotropic hormone and cortisol while electro-acupuncturing the points of Wangu and Taichong. *Liaoning J. Tradit. Chin. Med.* **34**(8), 1145–1146.

Yang, J., Yu, M. and Zhao, R. (1995) Influence of radiotherapy and chemotherapy on incretory function of malignant tumor patients and regulation function of acupuncture on it. *Acupunct. Res.* **20**(1), 1–4.

Section II
Common Practices

Chapter 5

A Practical Approach to Acupuncture

Abstract

Acupuncture is a practical maneuver used mainly for the control of pain resistant to conventional treatments and for the restoration of musculoskeletal functions after neurological damages. Acupuncture procedures initiate either complicated neurological activities at the spinal cord and or higher cerebral levels. Alternatively, indirect humoral stimulations affecting the overall bodily functions might be the result. At the present stage, such activities are demonstrated only qualitatively. Although the mechanisms of action are largely unknown, there are good reasons to support its use as an additional treatment option to conventional therapy.

Keywords: Acupuncture; Practical Approach; Traditional Theory.

5.1 Introduction

In 1997, the National Institutes of Health of US (NIH) held a consensus conference to work out a general policy towards the application of acupuncture in various areas of need. The conference organizers concluded that although many clinical studies failed to give solid evidence of efficacy when the fundamental principles of evidence based medicine are used as assessment tools, acupuncture's effects on the control of nausea and vomiting, pain of dental origin and under other circumstances are widely considered positive. Moreover, NIH were aware of the many physiological experiments being done on animals and humans, which are expected to be able to reveal the mechanisms of action sooner or later (NIH, 1997).

Since this important move taken by the NIH, the already rising popularity of acupuncture practice received further encouragement so that major hospitals in US, started to establish small acupuncture teams to take care of special needs. Some specialties like rehabilitation, rheumatology, psychiatry and oncology started to run integrated clinics in which acupuncture practice was always included. There is little doubt that, in US, Europe and within the wide territories of Chinese Communities, acupuncture is now the best known and most frequently used technique in alternative medicine (Birch and Kaptchuk, 1999).

As a matter of fact, the World Health Organization (WHO), in 1995, had already issued a users' guideline on the practice of acupuncture (Bannerman, 1979).

In the Chinese Communities, acupuncture naturally commands even a higher popularity. In China, acupuncture clinics are those dealing with the longest waiting lists in the public services of Chinese Medicine. In Hong Kong, patients suffering from chronic pain are constant customers. Neural deficits seldom recover completely: the sufferers most frequently seek acupuncturists' assistance (Wong *et al.*, 1993). Our service providers are aware of the need, such that acupuncture has become a well-accepted option among most hospital practitioners when the standard conventional treatment has failed to give satisfactory results.

This special issue of the Annals of Chinese Medicine aims at the provision of a comprehensive guide for all those using acupuncture as treatment options and also for some patients who like to understand more about the practice. Special chapters give guidelines to specific problems indicated for acupuncture, and would serve as practical references for the practicing acupuncturists about the indications, principles of treatment and practical applications.

The provision of information would not be useful without discussions about research and future development. In order to prepare for future studies, what is already known about the mechanisms of action must be reviewed. This introduction would therefore give the current knowledge about the physiological explanations about acupuncture and would also try to respond to some of the known difficulties and misunderstandings.

5.2 Some Accepted Theories on the Course of Events of Acupuncture

The WHO lists six categories of 36 health conditions that acupuncture is recommended to treat. They are problems of the upper respiratory tract, the respiratory system, gastrointestinal disorders, neurological and musculoskeletal disorders, and mouth and eye conditions. A Consensus Development Panel on Acupuncture of the NIH identified 11 conditions that can be effectively helped (NIH, 1997), and all these fall into the WHO list.

To justify such a large area of clinical applications, there must be sufficient evidence about the efficacy. If it takes time to unveil the mystery through research, there must be logical postulations or theories to explain the possible mechanisms of action. The following sections offer logical theories of explanation.

5.2.1 Traditional theory

A Chinese medicine practitioner will find no difficulty explaining the effects of acupuncture by referring to the concept of body *qi*. For him, the free flow of *qi* is the foundation of a balanced mind and body, i.e. a healthy person. Diseases are the products or indications of the interrupted flow of *qi* or the weakness of *qi*. The main function of acupuncture is to restore its free flow (Huangdi Neijing, 2010).

We do not yet have a suitable instrument that could be used to measure the level of *qi*. Thus, *qi* is considered to be a metaphysical understanding of the human body and its functions that does not have a scientific basis.

5.2.2 Pain control theory

The "gate theory" of Melzack and Wall has been used to explain what and how acupuncture does in the control of pain (Melzack and Wall, 1966). The pain stimulus sends a message up the spinal cord through the reticular formation in the brain stem to the thalamus. The message is then projected to diverse areas in the intermediate and higher brain. During the process of acupuncture another message is sent through a different tract in the spinal cord to various nuclei of the thalamus, then it is projected to various cortical areas of the higher brain. On its way to the thalamic nuclei, collaterals of the spinal thalamic tracts branch out and are projected to various levels of the brain stem and hypothalamus. Some of the descending neurons from the upper brain activate inhibitory inter-neurons, which in turn inhibit ascending pain signals. With acupuncture, this "gate" effect of pain message transmission is enhanced (Melzack *et al.*, 1977).

5.2.3 *High brain — neuro-humoral theory*

Scientists found that high brain, under the influence of acupuncture stimulation, sends out messages through beta-endorphin mechanisms (Han, 1995; He and Han, 1990). The neurotransmission channel related to peripheral stimulation activating a high brain signal which respond through a beta-endorphin mechanism has been worked out clearly in the explanation of milk production in a lactating mother. The baby feeding on the mother's breast stimulates tactile receptors, which send up messages via the spinal cord to the hypothalamus, thence to the pituitary which reactions through a neuro-humoral mechanism, sending oxytocin and prolactin into the blood circulation, thus maintaining the production of milk in the mammary glands.

Cho observed by using functional MRI, activation of higher brain areas such as visual and auditory cortices as a result of acupuncture. Signals from these areas might project through the limbic structures and descend to the hypothalamic centers to stimulate beta-endorphin secretion. The hypothesis goes one step further by describing the high brain messages reaching the hypothalamus directly or indirectly, then command the execution of endocrine, autonomic and other functions for the purpose of homeostasis. The pain control is only a small part of the much larger survival related functions of acupuncture disease treatment. Other functions include endocrine, autonomic and neurochemical activities mainly controlled by the hypothalamus, the central integrator and commanders of the brain and body (Cho *et al.*, 1998).

5.2.4 *Theories from the antagonists*

Antagonists against acupuncture are scientists who demand a perfect knowledge on the anatomical and physiological aspects of acupuncture before accepting it as a safe and trustworthy treatment procedure. Kim in North Korea declared in 1970 that he indentified anatomical structures along the acupuncture meridians which he described as small ducts like lymphatics, lined with cells named after himself as "Kim-bong corpuscles". However, the "ducts and corpuscles" have never been verified by other scientists who tried to repeat the anatomical and histological dissections (Soh K 2009). Since the late 1980s, many neurophysiology experiments have been completed to explore the neurological explanations to acupuncture. The results have been interesting but inconclusive. Antagonists therefore have preserved their antagonism and henceforth have labeled acupuncture as placebo-, suggestion- and stress-related phenomena.

(1) Placebo effects

Placebo is "an epithet given to any medicine adapted more to please than to benefit the patient". The fact is: all patients receiving treatment are expecting therapeutic effects. Factors unrelated to the treatment like the care expressed by the practitioner, the social contact during the consultation, and suggestions from the practitioner about the benefits of the treatment itself, will all be comforting to the patient. Placebo effects can be powerful, and this is why evidence-based medicine requires that all therapies should be measured against placebo control. Basically, placebo effects exist in every therapy, and acupuncture is not immune from this.

However, assuming acupuncture effects are pure placebo effects does not have strong support. Some important clinical observations strongly challenge the placebo theory. Acupuncture analgesia has been demonstrated in animals. Acupuncture effects are also achieved in children. Moreover, results from reviews of clinical trials on acupuncture for chronic pain suggested that placebo effects involved might reach within 30% of patients with chronic pain, while up to 70% of patients gained real pain controlling benefits (Pomeranz, 1989).

(2) Suggestion (hypnosis) effects

Acupuncture procedures have been assumed to be due to some form of positive suggestion, or hypnosis induced by the practitioner. This view could hardly stand for the following reasons: (i) acupuncture effects are achieved while the patients are wide awake and they could be engaged in active conversations, which will not happen in hypnotized patients (Melzack, 1975); (ii) psychophysical studies in humans have demonstrated that both good and poor respondents for hypnosis gained equal acupuncture benefits (Ulett, 1989); and (iii) acupuncture works in some live animals.

(3) Stress reactions

When people are in stressful conditions, for example, when running for their lives or competing for championship their pain threshold is markedly increased. This is called stress-induced analgesia. Acupuncture does not initiate sufficient stress to attain stress analgesia although stress may be produced by the needling procedure. A psychophysical study has shown that subjects who achieved good acupuncture responses are not more anxious than those who did not (Zaretsky *et al.*, 1976).

5.3 Auricular Acupuncture — What is Its Mechanism[1]

Like foot reflexology and hand and scalp acupuncture, auricular acupuncture is one of the mini-acupuncture systems that is based on the theory of holographic homunculus pattern. Since Paul Nogier of Lyon, France described his inverted fetus map, auricular acupuncture has been developed and widely applied in China.

Nogier thought that there are three different zones on the auricle that are related to different types of neural innervation related to different categories of embryological tissues (Nogier, 1983), and there is a special somatotopic organization of the acupoints on the auricle. The central concha of the auricle is innervated by the vagus nerve and serves as the region for autonomic regulation of pain and pathology produced from internal organs. The surrounding antihelix and antitragus ridges of the auricle represent somatic areas related to myofascial pain, back pain and headaches. The outer helix tail and earlobe represent the spinal cord and trigeminal neuralgia.

It has been known that there are both descending pain facilitation and descending pain inhibition systems in the central nervous system. Oleson

---

[1] This section is contributed by Dr. B. Xin, Beijing Centre for Acupuncture, Beijing, China.

proposed that the relief of pain by auricular acupuncture could be interpreted by the theory of stimulation-produced analgesia. The most potent area for obtaining stimulation-produced analgesia in rats is the midbrain periaqueductal gray area, which is a region containing neurons specifically responsive to noxious stimuli. For higher species, deep brain stimulation in the subcortical thalamus is a more potent site for stimulation-produced analgesia. Similar results have been found in human patients (Hsieh *et al.*, 1995). Positron emission tomography (PET) scan activity in the periaqueductal gray, hypothalamus, somatosensory cortex and prefrontal cortex can be activated by nociceptive pain messages. (Oleson *et al.*, 1980)

In order to examine the bioelectric properties of auricular acupoints, Oleson conducted a double-blind assessment in which 40 patients with specific musculoskeletal pain were recruited (Lao, 1996). The medical diagnosis was established through proper clinical investigations. Then a doctor with extensive auricular acupuncture knowledge examined the patient's ear without communicating with the patient. The painful auricular areas were found equivalent to the parts of the body where there was musculoskeletal pain. The overall accuracy rate was 75.2%. All these supported the fact that specific areas of the ear are related to specific parts of the body. Another assessment had been conducted to examine the correspondence of heart diseases to the inferior concha and tragus (auricular acupoint related to heart). Compared with the control group of healthy subjects (11%), the problem group had 84% of correlation in the inferior concha and 59% in the tragus.

5.4 Clinical Trials on Acupuncture

While the basic requirements for clinical trials on newly introduced pharmaceuticals have been widely adopted and follow a direction of three phases: phase I for safety, phase II for dosage, and phase III for efficacy. Clinicians might insist on this approach as universal requirements before a treatment regime is considered appropriate. We could apply the same procedures for the assessment of the clinical use of acupuncture.

Phase I trials aim at the establishment of the basic safety of a selected dosage delivered to the condition under investigation. These trials are generally of small sample sizes with no control groups. Several questions need to be answered during this phase when acupuncture is being investigated. The first question is whether standardized or individualized acupuncture will be suitable for the study, and the answer depends on the conditions being tested. If the patients share the same conventional or Chinese Medicine diagnoses, in other words, the patients belong to a homogeneous population, a design of standardized acupuncture is a good choice. On the contrary, individualized acupuncture will be more suitable for heterogeneous populations where many symptoms are divergent and different symptoms are being treated together. Therefore, the demand on the experience of the acupuncturist is much higher for individualized acupuncture than for formulated acupuncture. A wide range of literature needs to be reviewed and careful clinical observations are essential. With regard to the total duration and frequency of treatments, it is not easy to find the answer from the literature. Frequent assessments to check the changes of improvement are necessary in order to determine the frequency and duration of standardized or individualized treatment.

Compared with phase I, a control group should be applied in phase II. In this stage, the dose and safety are further confirmed and the preliminary information on the efficacy is also revealed. It is commonly recognized that designing a suitable control methodology for a certain study is a really difficult task for investigators. Currently, there are several control designs being used in clinical trials of acupuncture, including no treatment as control, sham acupuncture, placebo acupuncture, etc. All of them have disadvantages. Ideally placebo acupuncture, for example, helps to explain whether or not the effects of true acupuncture is due to placebo effect. But in actual practice a placebo design does not completely resemble the true acupuncture, and the patients will be fully aware of the different nature of practice (Witt *et al.*, 2006; Lai, 2001; Leung, 2003).

Phase III trials require a large population deduced from a statistical estimation according to an expected percentage of positive effects. Evidence-based medicine insists on randomization of assignments to the treatment and placebo group and double-blinding for both the recipients and assessors is much preferred. However, one should be skeptical whether true blinding is possible at all.

The three phases of clinical trials have been accepted as golden rules to the efficacy assessment for new drugs. It is obvious that these golden rules might not be suitable for acupuncture practice. Nevertheless, modern practitioners do not have an alternative method of assessment for efficacy. The widely accepted methodology, therefore, remains the only recognized approach on the proof of efficacy (Leung and Zhang, 2008).

For the acupuncture practitioner, however, experience and observations are more important than proper trials.

It has been observed in clinical practices that acupuncture works better for problems related to peripheral nerves and muscles, and displays better results in vascular diseases and post-operative rehabilitations. Other impressive results have been observed in facial paralysis, headache, trigeminal neuralgia, chronic low back pain, stroke rehabilitation, and some special areas, like bed-wetting in children, nausea and vomiting associated with pregnancy, and menstruation disorders. The postulation is that acupuncture helps to regulate the nerve-endocrine immunological circuit, when no obvious organic pathology exists.

Whatever is the situation, clinical trials for the efficacy of acupuncture performed for certain specific conditions are needed to establish wider recommendations and more reliable. Like all clinical trials, improvements in clinical symptoms and signs are the only fundamental requirements. Additional objective data like serological markers or images in special investigations are also helpful. Now that magnetic resonance and positron emission images could help identifying delicate changes in the soft tissues, from molecular reactions to oxygen contents, the changes can be recorded, analyzed, and be accepted as objective parameters of results of treatment. However, up to the present, special image changes remain experimental in the exploration of the neurological basis of acupuncture. It would be quite some time before these new sophisticated investigations could be proven practical assessment tools for the old technique of acupuncture.

5.5 Complications and Adverse Events in Acupuncture

Complications of life-threatening magnitude have been reported during and after acupuncture. These events are related to direct injuries to organs like the lungs and liver. In the former case, pneumothorax is caused by puncture of the pleura and in the latter, puncturing the liver results in hemoperitoneum. Such serious complications are real injuries imposed through careless maneuvers (Bhatt, 1985).

The Institute of Chinese Medicine at The Chinese University of Hong Kong has conducted research programs on acupuncture efficacy and clinical trials using acupuncture. Acupuncture clinical trials have been planned using a uniform set of acupuncture points for the treatment of clinical syndromes suffered by patients selected according to uniform criteria. The method of puncture, i.e. needle entry, depth reached, needling maneuvers, duration of needling, needle removal, and the use of electrical stimulation (where applied), were all standardized.

The patients who received acupuncture were recruited specifically for clinical trials on the following conditions: low back pain, paraplegia, failed back surgery syndrome, nocturnal enuresis, erectile dysfunction, migraine, nerve damage, hypertension, rheumatoid arthritis, overactive bladder in women, post-stroke rehabilitation, and postpartum depression. Patients with bleeding tendency and those maintained on anticoagulants were excluded (Vickers, 1996; Wu *et al.*, 2002).

All the treatments were performed by two highly qualified, experienced acupuncture specialists. The acupuncture treatments used for the different studies are summarized in Table 5.1. Adverse events and complications were specially monitored and recorded. A checklist of possible complications and adverse events of acupuncture (such as pneumothorax, nerve damage, obvious tissue or organ damage, bleeding, dizziness, fainting) was used by the two acupuncturists in a special investigation on adverse events. The two acupuncturists recorded all adverse effects during and after the treatment, and actively enquired about adverse feelings during the subsequent visit. Repetitions of adverse events in the same patient were considered separate incidents. All adverse reports were correlated with the disease condition, the acupuncture sites, depths of entry, and the body build of the patients.

From June 2002 to March 2005, a total of 2000 consecutive acupuncture treatments in 254 patients were given in a total of 11 projects. A total of eight cases of bleeding were recorded, six of which occurred in the hand. No other adverse events were reported.

Table 5.1. Acupuncture points used in the clinical studies described.

Condition	Points used
Failed back syndrome (using EA)	*Huatuo Jiaji* (EX-B-2, levels L2 to L5), BL40, BL60
Failed back syndrome (using manual stimulation)	BL23, BL26, GV4, KI3
Nocturnal enuresis	BL23, BL32, KI3, GV20, CV6, CV4, ST36, SP6
Erectile dysfunction	BL23, CV4, BL32, KI2, LR5, SP6
Migraine	GB20, GV20, *Taiyang* (EX-HN-5), GB8, LR3
Spinal cord damage	*Huatuo Jiaji* (EX-B-2, lumbar 2-5), GV4, BL62 Auricular points: *Shenmen*, Kidney, Vertebrae
Hypertension	ST36, LR3, GB20, LI11, SP6
Rheumatoid arthritis	LI11, TE5, LI4, ST36, GB34, GB39
Overactive bladder in women	GV20, BL26, BL28, BL32, SP6
Post-stroke rehabilitation	LI11, LI4, LI15, ST36, ST40, LR3 Scalp points: MS5, MS8, MS9
Postpartum depression	GV20, *Yintang* (EX-HN-3), CV6, ST36, SP6

None of the points used was near the thorax, thus avoiding any risk of the most common serious adverse event — pneumothorax (Leung, 2009). While acupuncture treatment should not be assumed to be always safe, complications causing real harm must be the result of negligence, which should be avoidable. A group of acupuncture experts in China had seriously looked into all possible adverse events that might occur during acupuncture and their report also showed that, by carefully controlling the setting and by using expert practitioners with carefully planned procedures in anatomically safe sites, adverse events could be reduced to an absolute minimum, and will consist solely of bleeding only.

One commonly described feeling among patients receiving acupuncture is "fainting" or "dizziness". Although postulations related to the meridian theory have been made, a more likely cause of this "adverse event" is a vago-vasal type of transient cerebral ischemia secondary to the sharp pain felt at the puncture site (Leung, 2009).

5.6 Difficulties with Acupuncture Research

Before more physiological evidences of the mechanism of action of acupuncture are available, difficulties related to acupuncture research would persist. The difficulties include the following:

5.6.1 Using placebo punctures

Placebo punctures have been tried under the following circumstances:
(1) puncturing at a short distance (1–1.5 cm) away from the selected meridian and acupoints;
(2) puncturing at another selected point known to be unrelated to the selected meridian;
(3) touching on the selected acupoint, then immediate withdrawal; and
(4) Using a special acupuncture needle with a rebound mechanism which facilitates the withdrawal (Witt *et al.*, 2006).

All these attempts would not be perfect choices. The recipient patients would be able to differentiate the different puncture sites. They would also be able to identify brief sharp touches and withdrawals with or without special devices.

When electrical stimulation is used as enforcement measures, placebo arrangement becomes absolutely meaningless. In actuality, the classical practice of acupuncture would not allow placebo arrangement. The essential requirement during the puncturing procedure includes the feeling of "*de-qi*", which is a very special sensory perception between pain and soreness. To achieve *de-qi* feeling, a substantial depth of puncture, together with manual rotation or vertical pushes are required. Such maneuvers will certainly allow the recipient to realize which puncture is real and which is sham. For the best results of acupuncture, the performer has to check with the recipient that the *de-qi* feeling is experienced before the needle is retained at the acupoint. Otherwise, a repeated puncture, possible at a different site is performed.

5.6.2 Standardized puncture treatment

In the classical acupuncture, the acupuncturist gives a comprehensive analysis of the symptom complex of the patient before deciding on the meridian and acupuncture points for treatment. Since the symptom complex tends to change with time and progress of the clinical condition, he has to flexibly change his plan of puncture according to the needs of the patient. Individualized puncture protocol is therefore one of the fundamental requirements of effective and efficient acupuncture treatment. However, a changing individualized protocol is unsuitable for clinical trials.

With these fundamental requirements, one has to realize that strict adherence to the rules of randomized control trials in evidence based practice is not possible for acupuncture research.

5.6.3 *Objective assessment of response*

All clinical efficacies should be assessed with as many objective means as possible. The main indications for acupuncture are pain control and neuromuscular rehabilitation, and both areas are deficient of perfect objective measurement tools. The reliance on subjective reports will persist and would continuously invite criticism and skepticism from the antagonists.

5.7 Conclusions

Acupuncture procedures obviously initiate either complicated neurological activities at the spinal cord and higher cerebral levels, or indirect humoral stimulations affecting the overall bodily functions. At present, such activities are demonstrated only qualitatively. No detailed knowledge about the exact channels of activities are yet known. The mechanisms could be so complicated that it might take an extremely long time before the knowledge would be ready for practical utilization.

Acupuncture is a practical maneuver for the control of chronic pain resistant to conventional treatment and for the restoration of musculoskeletal functions after neurological damage. Although the mechanisms of action are not yet known thoroughly, there are good reasons to support its use as an additional treatment option to conventional therapy.

References

Bannerman, R.H. (1979) *Acupuncture: The World Health Organization View.* World Health Organization, Geneva.

Bhatt. Sanders, D. (1985) Acupuncture for rheumatoid arthritis: An analysis of the literature. Semin. *Arthritis. Rheum.* **14**(4), 225–231.

Birch, S. and Kaptchuk, T.J. (1999) History, Nature and current practice of acupuncture. In: *Acupuncture: A Scientific Appraisal.* (eds.) Ernst, E. and White, A. Butterworth Heinemann, Oxford, pp. 11–30.

Cho, Z.H., Chung, S.C. and Jones, J.P. (1998) New findings of the correlation between acupoints and corresponding brain cortices using functional MRI. *Proc. Natl. Acad. Sci. USA* **95**(5), 2670–2673.

Han, J.S. (1995) Cholecystokivein Octapeptide (CCK8), A negative feedback control mechanism for opiod analgesia. *Prof. Brain Res.* **105**, 263–271.

He, CM. and Han, J.S. (1990) Attenuation of low rather than high frequency electro-acupuncture analgesia by microinjection of B endorphin Antiserum into the periaqueductal gray in rats. *Acupunct. Sci. Int. J.* **1**, 94–99.

Hsieh, J., Stahle-Backdahl, M. Hagermark, O. and Stone-Elander, S. (1995) Traumatic nociceptive pain activates the hypothalamus and the periaqueductal gray: A positron emission tomography study. *Pain* **64**, 303–314.

Huangdi, N. (2010) Questions and Answers (Zu-run) Nai-jing, Chinese Classic. Ancient Chinese Medicine Press.

Lai, S.L, (2001) Clinical trials of Traditional Chinese Medicine. In: *Clinical Trials of Traditional Chinese Materia Medica.* Guangdong People's Publisher, China, chapters 2–4.

Lao, L. (1996) Acupuncture techniques and devices. *J. Altern Compl. Med.* **2**(1), 23–5.

Leung, P.C. (2003) Clinical trials using Chinese Medicine. In: *A Comprehensive Guide to Chinese Medicine.* World Scientific Publisher, Singapore.

Leung, P.C. and Zhang, L. (2008) Complications and adverse events in clinical trials of acupuncture. *Acupunct. Med.* **26**(2), 121–122.

Leung, P.-C. Zhang, L. and Cheng, K. (2009) Acupuncture: Complications are preventable not adverse events. *Clin. J. Integr. Med.* **15**(3), 229–232.

Melzack, R. (1975) How acupuncture can block pain. In: *Pain Clinical and Experimental Perspectives.* (ed.) Weisenberg, M. Mosby Company, Saint Louis.

Melzack, R. and Wall, P. (1966) *Peripheral Nerve and Spinal Mechanisms In the Challenge of Pain.* Penquin, London, pp. 81–107.

Melzack, R., Stillwell D. and Fox, E. (1977) Trigger points and acupuncture points for pain: correlations and implication. *Pain* **3**, 3–23.

National Institutes of Health Consensus Panel (1997) Acupuncture: NIH Consensus Development Conference Statement, Nov 3–5. **15**(5), 1–34.

Nogier, P. (1983) From Auriculotherapy to Auriculomedicine. Mainsonneuve, Moulins-les-Metz.

Kroening, R. and Oleson, T. (1985) Rapid narcotic detoxification in chronic pain patients treated with auricular electroacupuncture and naloxone. *Int. J. Additions* **20**(9), 1347–1360.

Oleson, T.D., Kroening, R.J. and Bresler, D.E. (1980) An experimental evaluation of auricular diagnosis: The somatotopic mapping of musculoskeletal pain at acupuncture points. *Pain* **8**, 217–229.

Pomeranz, B. (1989) Acupuncture analgesia for chronic pain: Brief survey of clinical trial. In: *Scientific Bases of Acupuncture.* (eds.) Pomeranz, B. and Stux, G. Springer-Verlag, Berlin, pp. 197–199.

Soh, K. (2009) Bonghan circulatory system as an extension of acupuncture meridians. *J. Acupunct. Meridian Stud.* **2**, 93–106.

Ulett, G. (1989) Studies supporting the concept of physiological acupuncture. In: *Scientific Bases of Acupuncture.* (eds.) Pomeranz, B. and Stux, G. Springer-Verlag, Berlin, pp. 177–196.

Vickers, A.J. (1996) Can acupuncture have specific effects on health? A systematic review *J. R. Soc. Med.* **89**, 303–311.

Witt, C.M., Jena, S. and Brinkhaus, B. (2006) Acupuncture in patients with osteoarthritis of the knee: A randomized controlled trial. *Arthritis and Rheum.* **54**(11), 3485–3493.

Wong, T.W., Wong, S.L. and Donnan, S. (1993) Traditional Chinese Medicine and Western Medicine in Hong Kong. *J. HK Med. Assoc.* **45**, 275–284.

Wu, Q., Huang, J. and Lai, X. (2002) Study on adverse events of acupuncture and moxibustion. *Chin. Acupunct. Moxibustion* **22**(5), 339–341.

Zaretsky, H.H., Lee, M.H., *et al.* (1976) Psychological factors and clinical observations in acupuncture analgesia and pain abatement. *J. Psychol.* **93**(1st Half), 113–120.

Chapter 6

Technique of Manual Puncturing

Abstract

No English word could be borrowed to carry the meaning of de-qi, which is a strange feeling between pain and numbness when the acupuncture needle reaches a certain depth down an acupoint and when manual manipulation of whirling, or thrusting is applied. This feeling indicates the right position in an effective maneuver. The word "acuesthesia" has been created for the sake of common understanding for de-qi. Acuesthesia and its relationship with the nervous system is complex. It is held that the "arrival of acuesthesia" is related to the peripheral nervous pathway, primarily manifested on the sensory (possibly proprioceptive) tracts, transmitting higher up to the central nervous system.

Keywords: Manual Puncturing; De-qi; Acuesthesia.

6.1 Description of Acuesthesia in Classic Medical Document

In *"Ling Shu: Condition of Evil Qi Fu Zang Disease"*, it says: "once the *qi* point was hit, the needle moves as if in a small house". In *"Zhen Jiu Da Cheng Volume 2: Biao You Fu"*, it says: "the arrival of *qi* is like fish struggling up and down after swallowing the hook, when *qi* does not arrive, it is like in the deep hollow of a secluded hall", "if feeling is light, smooth and slow, it means *qi* is yet to come, while sinking, rough and tight means *qi* appears". *"Yi Xue Ru Men"*: "When under the needle there is a heavy, tight and full feeling, *qi* has come, if under it the feeling is light and floating and empty moving, *qi* has not yet appeared". *"Zhen Jiu Da Cheng"*: "light floating, vacuity smooth, slow and late, if these three conditions are present after needle insertion, true *qi* has not arrived, with sink-heavy, rough-stagnate, tight-replete, the presence of these three means the right *qi* has come".

With regard to the description of acuesthesia, there are clinical experiments to explain it. For example, someone conducted a 1000-point time experiment on puncturing points to observe the conditions of acuesthesia, the results revealed that under the needle the sink-tight, sore, numb and distention sensations come out at the same time occupied 73.6%, with sink-tight but without sore, numb and distention sensations, 22.5%, with sore, numb and distention but without sink-tight sensations, 2.3%, others occupied 1.6%, so it was considered that "acuesthesia" could include sore, numb, distention sensations, and sore, numb and distention sensations might not be equivalent to acuesthesia. Whatever the case is, the sink-tight sensation under the needle may be accepted as acuesthesia (Liu, 1963).

6.2 Clinical Meaning of Acuesthesia

The clinical meaning of acuesthesia is recorded in various kinds of classical acupuncture documents. For example, *"Ling Shu: Nine Needle and 12 Sources"* states that "the essence of needling depends on getting the *qi* before it is effective", and Dou Han Qing of Ming Dynasty in his *"Biao You Fu"* says: "the quick arrival of *qi* gives rise to quick effect, the slow arrival of *qi* makes the case incurable". *"Zhen Jiu Da Cheng"* says: "when needling gets *qi* fast, disease is easy to heal and the effect is also fast; if *qi* arrives late, disease is difficult to heal with incurable anxiety". In *"Jin Zhen Fu"* and *"Biao You Fu"* there are also similar statements. Thus, whether there is acuesthesia would directly affect clinical treatment effect. Since ancient time, acuesthesia has been a needling effect demanded by clinical acupuncture practitioners.

Modern clinical studies also indicate that acuesthesia is closely related to effects of clinical treatment. For example, scientists conducted an experiment using the change of electrogastrol activity as an index of needling effect to compare the relationship between different acuesthesia states and needling effects by needling ST 36. The experiment adopted muscle injection of anticholinergic chloride 654–2 to inhibit electrogastrol activity, and the experiment data indicated that after injection of muscle with 654–2, it could produce the background of electrogastrol activity inhibition which is about 50% weaker than before the muscle injection. Right after the injection, needling was applied to bilateral ST 36. In the non-acuesthesia group, no manipulation was used after insertion of needle, which was kept loose.

For the acuesthesia group, after insertion of needle manipulation was carried out with even reinforcement and twirling of the needle for about 20 min was done every 5–10 min. In this group during the manipulation, the testees felt one or more of the sore, numb, distended or heavy sensations, and the operator also felt the heavy or hard repletion sensation. The electrogastrol changes of the acuesthesia group when compared with the control group, showed significant difference. In another group of experiment, observation was conducted on the influence of needling "PC 6" on Coronary heart disease (CHD) patient's heart function, which indicates that acuesthesia could achieve better clinical treatment effect (Hunag, 1999).

6.3 Method of Attaining Acuesthesia

Achieving acuesthesia has to be planned before needle insertion. To achieve the result of acuesthesia, the most basic requirement, of course, is the accuracy of point positioning. Besides, an accurate grasp of needling angle, direction and depth, plus a choice of appropriate needle manipulation need to be fulfilled. Other requirements include patience and good treatment environment. For the physically weak testee, needle should be retained to wait for *qi*, that means retaining needle in the point until *qi* arrives or use gentle lifting-thrusting and twirling-turning manipulation, taking advantage of supplementary flicking, handle scrapping or shaking to stimulate *qi* (Sun, 2002). There are also clinical reports on applying moxibustion to promote acuesthesia to appear (Yin *et al.*, 1983).

6.4 Studies on the Mechanism of Acuesthesia

The objective criteria of acuesthesia, and the local and whole body changes after acuesthesia, have greatly aroused clinicians' interest, leading to a large amount of clinical and laboratory explorations.

6.4.1 *The relationship between acuesthesia and puncture morphology*

(1) To study the structural basis of acuesthesia, an experiment was conducted on the domestic rabbits, using electromyography (EMG) as index and putting markers (blue dot) on the needle tip to observe

acuesthesia of rabbit's ST 36 in relation to the depth of puncture. Observations were made on 27 puncture when myoelectric expression was induced. The Blue dots mostly fell into muscles, or on the overlapping area of two muscle bundles. In the centre of these blue dots and in the surrounding 1.5 mm, the tissue structures included muscle fibers, a number of myelinated and amyelinated nerve fibers, small blood vessels, muscle spindles and lamellar corpuscles. It is therefore deducted that the structural basis of acuesthesia is multifocal, which could include various nerve endings, nerve receptor and blood vessels, and acuesthesia has no strict structural basis (Zeng *et al.*, 1982).

(2) There was a clinical observation which discovered that acuesthesia was closely related to the "sink-tight" sensation under the needle, and a further observation found that when there was acuesthesia felt on withdrawal of the needle, there was also the "sink-tight" sensation felt in three out of four acupuncture needles carried muscle fibers. It was presumed therefore that the muscle fibers twining could be the major factor leading to the "sink-tight" sensation of acuesthesia (Liu, 1963).

(3) One experiment using ultrasonic technique to observe the acuesthesia process was conducted. The results revealed the following: (i) when the needle tip was withdrawn up to the outer perimysium, acuesthesia occurred; (ii) when the needle tip reached the muscle, acuesthesia was weakened; (iii) if the needle tip stayed at the outer perimysium and stimulation was increased, acuesthesia feeling would be increased; and (iv) sometimes during acuesthesia, muscular fibers gliding could be observed. The experiment suggested that the occurrence of acuesthesia was related to the stimulation of outer perimysium and the gliding of muscular fibers (Shen *et al.*, 1995).

(4) Another experiment was conducted to detect if acuesthesia depths are affected by body types, namely fat, medium and thin body builds, as well as positions as the head, trunk, upper limbs and lower limbs. The results indicated that the depth of acuesthesia detected in the fat people group was deeper, and among the thin people group, the acuesthesia felt was shallower. The depth of acuesthesia from the head was shallow as compared with that from the trunk and four limbs. It was found at the same time that in testees who were nervous, and

hypersensitive, acuesthesia were shallower than the ordinary testees. Cancer and stroke patients felt acuesthesia deeper than ordinary testees (Lin *et al.*, 1994).

6.4.2 *Relationship between acuesthesia and electromyogram*

(1) When needling was applied to "ST 36" of the domestic rabbit so as to observe the relationship between acuesthesia and the changing position of the acupuncture needle using the electromyogram, it was formed that under normal circumstances, when sensation under the hand was "loose and empty", i.e. most often there was no firing of myo-electricity. If there was sensation, under the hand of a "sink-tight" sensation, there should be firing of myoelectricity.

(2) It was found that when there was no acuesthesia after needling, the acupuncturist's sensation under his hand appeared loose and weak, and the testee had no sore, numb, heavy and distended sensation, no emitted, basically there was no change in myoelectric signal occurred before and after needling. However, under the circumstances of acuesthesia, if the testee had a sore, numb, heavy and distended sensation, while the acupuncturist had the sink-tight sensation under his hand; at the point location, a myoelectric signal was emitted, and such signal was different from interference emitted by active muscle movement. In the test, it was also observed that this kind of point myoelectric signal has a parallel relationship with needle sensation; whenever the needle sensation was strong, the amplitude of point myoelectric signal emission and the number of occurrences would also increase (Liu *et al.*, 2005).

6.4.3 *The relationship between acuesthesia and nervous system*

(1) An experiment was conducted on human volunteers, using electrical stimulation on human body PC 6, and simultaneously the recording electrol response induced by stimulating PC 3 on the Pericardium Meridian in an attempt to explore any transmission between the two points. The experiment was conducted on 25 adults (including six spinal tetraplegics). The stimulating pulse was in direct flow square

wave form, with wave length of 0.5 ms, frequency at 1 Hz, intensity was limited within testees' endurance, guided by bipolar needle electrodes, and the electrol response induced by the stimulation through the AC amplifier was input into an adder. After intensifying 50–500 times, memory was used to display waves, and an analysis of the electrol response within 409.5 m/s after triggering was carried out. When needling PC 6, the testees' main complaint was mostly sore and distention sensation. After providing electrical pulses, most of their sensation turned numb and distended or sore, with jerking of the thumbs and forefingers. At this time, the electrol response of transmission speed of 55–78 m/s could be measured, and after increasing the strength, seven volunteers still maintain electrol response of transmission of 42–52 m/s. Those with spinal tetraplegia and upper limbs anesthesia could accept much stronger electro stimulation than a normal person (Meridian Acupuncture Anaesthesia Research room Unit 1, Shanghai CTM Research Institute, 1977).

(2) Another experiment was conducted on 16 normal persons in which needling was applied to their PC 6. After generating the sore, distended and heavy sensation, they were given square wave electrostimulation with wave length of 0.1–0.5 ms, frequency at 1–10 Hz, and with the adjustment of voltage strength to generate certain needle competence response after which blood flow of the upper arm was blocked; after 10 min, an observation was made every 2 min on the skin area of PC 6 to see its response to touching and pressure pain stimulation. When the touch of Electro-Acupuncture (EA) competence had entirely disappeared, manual needling with lifting-thrusting, twirling-turning stimulation on PC 6 was subsequently applied, and the time when the manual needling sensation disappeared was recorded. The results indicated that after blocking blood flow of the upper arm, it was the pericardial meridian puncture which disappeared with touch and pressure sensation, while the time of disappearance of manual needling sensation often coincided with that of pain sensation. It is inferred that the transmission message given through EA and manual needling depends on different mechanisms. For EA it is primarily through the thick nerve fibers, while manual needling excites small nerve fibers (Meridian Acupuncture

Anaesthesia Research room Unit 1, Shanghai CTM Research Institute, 1977).

(3) A study made use of patients suffering from syringomyelia, which affected pain and temperature sensation. Needling was applied to 37 cases of syringomyelia, 20 cases of neuropathy such as spinal cord transection, 20 healthy persons (LI 10, LI 4 and ST 36, etc.), to observe their needling sensation. The results showed that for: (i) 56 cases when treated with normal needling and twirling, the needling sensation was primarily distension 91.07%, sore 41.07%, numb 33.93%, heavy 14.28%, and transmission 58.93%; (ii) seven cases of syringomyelia patients who could not detect pain and temperature also did not feel anything when their LI 10 was punctured, 30 cases whose pain and warm sensation were only weakened felt a needling sensation, pain and warm sensation, all of which are related to spinothalamic tracts; and (iii) 20 cases of spinal cord transaction patients lost their needling sensation, suggesting that the needling sensation is related to normal nervous path (Meridian Acupuncture Anesthesia Theory Study Group, Shandong Medical College, 1977).

6.5 Conclusions

It could be concluded that:

(1) Regarding the anatomical foundation that generates acuesthesia, conclusions are varied and controversial. The most likely tissues responsible probably exist in the muscle layer. It has observed found that twining muscle fibers produced a feeling closely related to acuesthesia. There were also results showing that on the contrary, needling reaching the muscle layer could produce weak feelings, and the best needling sensation was found when the needle just reached the external perimysium. Other maintained that acuesthesia could be involving the nerve endings, receptors and the nervous structure of vascular wall.

(2) The relationship between acuesthesia and electromyogram is reaching a basic consensus, i.e. acuesthesia is related to electromyographic changes of the punctured muscle.

(3) Acuesthesia and its relationship with the nervous system is complex and complicated. Basically it is held that the "arrival of acuesthesia"

is related to the peripheral nervous pathway, primarily manifested on the sensory (deep pain sensation and temperature sensation) tracts, transmitting higher up to central nervous system.

References

Huang, X. (1999) The initial observation of the relationship of arrival of *qi* (*deqi*) with the needle efficiency. *Chin. Acupunct. Moxibustion* **1**, 19–21.

Lin, Z., Wang, Q., Huang, Z., *et al.* (1994) Study on depth of getting *qi* in clinical practice. *Chin. J. Integr. Tradit. West. Med.* **14**(2), 94–96.

Liu, Y. (1963) Preliminary exploration of acupuncture *Deqi* and feel of tingling swelling. *Shanghai J. Acupunct. Moxibustion* **1**, 24–26, 8.

Liu, Z., Yin, T., Guan, X., *et al.* (2005) Primary study on objective evaluation parameter and method of acupuncture deqi and maneuver. *Chin. J. Clin. Rehabil.* **9**(29), 119–121.

Meridian acupuncture anesthesia principle research group of Shandong Medical College (1977) Observation of acupuncture "deqi" principle and the pathway on syringomyelia patients and healthy people. Acupunct. Res. **z1**, 14.

Meridians acupuncture anesthesia research team one of Shanghai institute of Chinese medicine. (1977) Physiological observation of the human acupoint acupuncture ¾ effects of blocking the upper arm blood line on the electric acupuncture sensation and manual acupuncture sensation. *Acupunct. Res.* **z1**, 12.

Meridians acupuncture anesthesia research team, Shanghai institute of Chinese medicine (1977) Morphological observation of the human acupoint acupuncture sensation. *Acupunct. Res.* **z1**, 12.

Shen, Z. and Chen, D. (1995) Ultrasonic applications in acupuncture medicine (2nd Report), Using ring probe to observe the sites of "*deqi*". *Foreign Med. Sci.* **17**(3), 53–54.

Sun, G. (2002) *Zhenjiuxue. (Acupuncture and Moxibustion).* People's Medical Publishing House, pp. 514–515.

Yin, K. and Jiao, X. (1983) Some experiences and ways to promote acupuncture arrival of *qi* (*deqi*) *J. Tradit. Chin. Med.* **4**, 51.

Zeng, Z., Xu, M. and Dai, J. (1982) Rabbit acupuncture "arrival of *qi* (*deqi*)" and point tissue structure observation. *Shanghai J. Acupunct. Moxibustion* **3**, 12–15.

Chapter 7

Acupuncture for Headache

Abstract

Migraine is a recurrent seizure of vascular headache, which is common, especially among females. The headache may happen on one side or both sides of the head, frequently accompanied with nausea and vomit. The exact pathogenesis of migraine is still unclear. It could be related to the following factors: intracranial abnormal arterial responses to systolic and diastolic pulse waves; loss of balance in active vascular humoral substances, such as a decrease of 5-HT, or an increase of substance P and neurokinin, a pain inducing substance; or decreasing release of β-endorphin, etc. Migraine belongs to the category of "headache" and "head wind" in Chinese medicine. Current treatment of migraine primarily relies on ergotamine derivatives, such as caffeine, ergotamine, and 5-HT inhibitor, β-blocker, levodopa, etc. The immediate effects of acupuncture treatment could be remarkable for migraine and angioneurotic headache.

Keywords: Migraine; Headache; Acupuncture; and Moxibustion.

7.1 Acupuncture Method

One of the characteristics of acupuncture treatment of migraine is the selection of points by different meridians related to the headache. Take for example, if headache is on the *Yangming* Meridian, viz. on the eyebrow ridge, ST 8, LI 4 and EX-HN3 (*Yintang*) are selected. For a headache on the *Taiyang* Meridian, viz. on the posterior occiput down to the neck, SI 3, GV 16, GB 20 and BL10 are selected. For a headache on the *Shaoyang* Meridian, viz. ache on the temple and skull region, GB 8, TE 17, TE 5 and GB 41 are selected. For a headache on the *Jueyin* Meridian, viz. top of the head and linked to the eye system, GV 20, EX-HN1, PC 6, and LR 3 are selected. In clinical study conducted to treat 108 cases, full recovery (symptoms totally disappeared, no seizure in a half-year follow-up period) was 54.63% significantly effective (ache significantly reduced) was 25.93%, turning better (ache reduced with number of seizure reduced) was 12.96%. It was also observed that those patients with less than half a year's history did best, whereas those with more than three years' history had a poorer response, and with high recurrent rate (Xing, 1995).

(1) A clinical study was done to compare medicinal treatment using pizotyline with acupuncture. The results showed that the full recovery rate and effective rate of the acupuncture group were 48.7% and 92.1%, significantly higher than those of medicine group (22.0%, 76.0%) (Liu *et al.*, 2002).

(2) Another study using Sumatriptan succinate as the control group for the treatment of acute seizures of migraine. The results showed that after treatment for 0.5 hour, the acupuncture group's effective rate was significantly higher than that of medicine group (82.35%, 35.71%), and treatment after two hours, the acupuncture group and medicine groups became similar in their effective rate (88.24%, 78.57%) (Yu *et al.*, 2000).

(3) One study using primarily acupoints designated to the function of mental tranquility for migraine selected HT 7, EX-HN 1, EX-HN 5, and GV 20. Treatment course lasted six days, and in between courses, two resting days were allowed. Acupuncture was carried out for two treatment courses and after six months an evaluation of the treatment effect was made. The total effectives rate was 96.6%; at the same time, observations were made on the patient's cerebrovascular blood resistance and its elasticity changes. It was found that after acupuncture, the patient's vascular pulsatility index (PI) and resistive index (RI) were significantly lowered, suggesting that acupuncture applied on the points of tranquility, could achieve the additional balance of intracranial vascular blood flow (Gu, 2005).

(4) Some acupuncture experts selected acupoint according to the *yin-yang* states of bodily function, and acupuncture was applied for ten days as one treatment course, allowing 2–3 resting days in between the

courses. The results showed a total effectives rate of 93.2% (Yuan *et al.*, 2004).

(5) The joined acupuncture technique was employed, using one needle to reach two points. In one study, 90 cases of migraine patients were randomly divided into the joined puncture group and the normal acupuncture group. The point selected for the joined puncture group was as follows: EX-HN 5 joined with GB 8, GB 15 joined with GB 17, GV 23 joined with GV 20, GB 19 joined with GB 20, LI 4 joined with SI 3. For the joined punctures, needles were inserted for a depth of 40–50 mm, with rapid, small range twirling turns lasting for 1 min and the needles were retained for 30 min. For the control group, the selection followed the head-wind stasis principle, viz. ashi point, LI 4, SP 6, BL 17, and BL 40. The results showed: (i) the total effectivene rate of the treatment group was 97.8%, significantly better than control group's 80.0%; (ii) both groups significantly improved patients' number of headache seizure, headache severity, duration and accompanied symptoms. The treatment group appeared better than the control group; and (iii) both groups significantly improve patients' middle cerebral artery (MCA), anterior cerebral artery (ACA) and posterior cerebral artery (PCA) blood flow speed during the headache period.

7.2 Moxibustion

Moxibustion could provide warming and speeding effect of acupuncture. A study examined the acupuncture of GB 20 and TE 5 together with a 1.5 cm moxa stick placed on the needle handles for warming moxi-acupuncture once daily for ten days as a treatment course. The results indicated that warming acumoxi could significantly increase patients' cerebral blood flow, average blood flow speed, and enlarge vertebrobasilar internal diameter; it could also lower blood viscosity, increase the saturation of oxygen in cerebral tissues, lower blood platelet 5-HT, and raise the level of 5-HT in plasma (Wang, 2004).

In other clinical reports using warming moxiacupuncture significant lowering of serum thromboxane and epoprostenol of middle-aged and senior patients suffering from persistent migraine were shown (Zhu *et al.*, 1999).

7.3 Electro-Acupuncture (EA) Treatment

(1) There was a report of multi-centre randomized controlled trial in which 300 cases of migraine patients were randomly divided into a treatment group and a control group, each with 150 cases. They were given EA treatment on EX-HN 5, or oral anti-migraine drug as control. Observations were made before and after treatment on headache severity score, degree of relief, and frequency of headache. Treatment was carried out once daily over five days as a treatment course, with a total of four courses, and a break of two days in between courses. For the medicinal group: two Somedon were given, three times daily, together with ergotamine caffeine, two tablets and diazepam, 2.5 mg, three times daily. Treatment course was the same as the EA group. Both groups of patients after EA or medicine showed a declining headache intensity that was more significant in the EA than the control group. Comfort time was 388.6 ± 430.1 min in the EA group and 163.3 ± 182.3 min in the medicine group. The relief rate was 80.1% and 76.4% respectively, for the EA and medicine group ($p > 0.05$).

(2) Another study was carried out to examine the treatment effect of EA on migraine by applying it to GB 40, making use of multi-centre, randomized controlled research method, and taking ST 25 as the control. It was found that simply applying EA to GB 40 has a better treatment effect. Cyclic analgesic effect was evaluated in terms of headache severity, duration, recurrence, accompanied symptoms, and plasma 5-HT value. Results showed that there was no significant difference between the two groups in terms of immediate analgesic effects. However after treatment for four weeks, three months, and six months, the treatment group was significantly better than the control group. The 5-HT level of the treatment group was significantly higher than that of control group (Jia *et al.*, 2004).

7.4 Tap Acupuncture

(1) This is a method to treat migraine by using a "plum-blossom needle" to tap-along the Gallbladder Meridian and *Shaoyang* and Bladder

Meridian of the Foot, as well as *Taiyang* Meridian, which runs along the head. In case of severe headache, tapping could be made to produce slight bleeding. Such needling was done once daily for five days as a treatment course. The results showed that out of 56 cases of migraine patients, 45 were cured, 11 cases became better, and the overall response rate was 80.36% (Yang *et al.*, 2000).

(2) The ashi point is another acupuncture position where tap acupuncture is to be applied. The migraine site was sterilized, then the acupuncturist used the edge of his right palm and ring and, little fingers to tap the painful site before starting needle tapping. Tapping 200 times would relieve the headache. The cure rate could reach 68.6% (Zhang *et al.*, 1988).

(3) One study used a "7-star needle" for tap needling on the GV and Bladder Meridian, on the back of the patient from GV 20 to GV 1 and Bladder Meridian of Foot-*Taiyang*, from BL11 to BL 54, 1.5 cun lateral to the spine. Tapping was applied until skin became red, once every other day, for ten days as a treatment course, with 2–3 resting days in between courses. For the control group, bilateral GB 1, GB 20, LR 3 and EX-HN 3 were selected with routine acupuncture. The tap acupuncture (80%, 95%) was found to have better results than the routine acupuncture group (50%, 85.3%) (Li, 1997).

7.5 Using Three-Edged Needles

(1) Three-edged needles are thought to have the merit of opening up the orifices and discharging heat, speeding up circulation and dispelling stasis, and is suitable for migraine treatment. In one study, 122 cases of migraine patients were randomly divided into three-edged needle group and routine treatment group (each with 61 cases). For the three-edged needle group: acupoints selected were GV 23, GV 21, GV 20, GV 18, and GV 17. They could be supplemented with GB 20, GB 12, BL 10, and all points on the head were needled with the pecking method until a slight oozing of blood appeared. The results showed that the three-edged needle group, achieved a higher effective rate (95.08%) compared with the routine acupuncture group (91.80%).

(2) Other clinical observations using the three-edged needle to puncture as well as introduce bleeding showed similarly better results. The major points selected were EX-HN 5, LU 5. After routine sterilization, a sharp three-edged needle was used to puncture the corresponding spots to a depth of 2–5 mm, and 5–10 ml of blood were let out from each acupoint. Treatment was carried out every ten days, and three treatment sessions were recommended as a course. Comparing with standard acupuncture on EX-HN 5, GV 20 and GB 8, the results revealed that the immediate and late effects of the three-edged needle blood-letting group were better than the routine acupuncture group (Wang *et al.*, 2002).

7.6 Acupoint Injection

(1) Acupoint injection achieves the dual effect of needling and medication. In reports on treating migraine with acupoint injection, the medicinal material injected included usually hormones, vitamins and herbal extracts. One reported the injection of metacortandralone to point SI 17 and/or EX-HN 5, GB 20, plus the ashi point. In the 105 migraine patients that were studied, 83.3% pain stopped at initial treatment on follow-up visit 6–18 months later, and only 3.8% had recurrent seizures after three months, which responded well to repetition of treatment (Li *et al.*, 1991).

(2) Another report used Vitamin B1 to inject EX-HN 5, GB 20, ST 8, LI 4 for 50 migraine patients. One treatment course of ten sessions gain a total effectives rate of 94%, better than simple acupuncture treatment (40 cases) (Cui *et al.*, 2005).

(3) There was another report on the use of herbal extracts of dalbergia and salvia to treat 100 migraine patients. The points selected were BL 40, GB 34, and the injection was given every other day. Sixty-two cases were cured with this treatment, which resulted in a total effective rate of 94%; better than traditional EA treatment (82%) (Liu *et al.*, 2003).

7.7 Summary and Discussion

Migraine belongs to the category of "headache" and "head wind" in TCM. The disease is mainly manifested as "wind", "phlegm", and "stasis", etc.

The characteristics of headache is the on and off seizure from time to time, the longer the duration, the more difficult the cure. The immediate effects of acupuncture treatment on migraine is remarkable, and long term results are also improved.

A acupuncture and moxibustion treatment of migraine demands a careful selection of acupoints which includes the following:

(1) Use of ashi point. For migraine patients who have obvious tender spots on the head, those points (i.e. ashi points) are most favourable for acupuncture treatment. Energetic manipulation on those points gives great benefits after which the needle could be withdrawn without the need for retention. Normally 1-3 tender spots are selected for treatment.

(2) Selection of head points. There are two ways to select head points: one is the traditional head transport point, mainly based on headache position to divide the meridian in selecting points, that means the meridian characteristics of the headache position could guide the selection on the corresponding meridians for acupuncture. For example, for *Yangming* Meridian headache (pain on the eyebrow) select ST 8, EX-HN 3. For *Taiyang* Meridian headache (pain on the back of occipital down the neck) select CV 16, GB 20, BL10. For *Shaoyin* Meridian headache (pain on bilateral temple regions) select GB 8, TE 17. For *Jueyin* Meridian headache (pain on the top together with the eye system) select ashi, GV 20, EX-HN 1.

(3) For migraine treatment, acupoints on lower limbs could also be selected. For example, the points commonly used are LR 3, GB 41, KI 11.

(4) Point has been done according to the special diagnostic feeling of the acupuncturist, taking reference to the wellbeing of liver, blood kidney or digestive activities.

7.8 Additional Views

Headaches are a common ailment. The usual presentations frequently enjoy spontaneous control and simple analgesic medication could be very effective. Alternative treatment like acupuncture, therefore, is necessary only under special circumstances.

Under special circumstances, however, like chronic recurrent migraine, or more rarely, trigeminal neuralgia, in spite of specialist treatment, pain still occurs regularly. Acupuncture could be indicated to either induce a quicker control when the attack comes, or to make the recurrences less frequent. Acupuncture for resistant migraine and trigeminal neuralgia could produce quick responses, however, a dramatic cure is still be exceptional.

7.8.1 *Migraine*

Two special techniques are commonly used for the control of migraine.

(1) "Speedy needling"
On the acupoint is selected, the needle is introduced quickly through the skin surface at a slanting angle so that the depth is only 1–2 cm. Manipulation of the needle needs to be quick and repetitive with an aim of initiating sharp "soaring feelings".
(2) "Lazy needling"
After introducing the needle like just described under "speedy needling", the needle is firmly pinched between two fingers which direct the distal end of the needle on a repeated up-and-down movement. The aim is to initiate as much soaring feeling as possible. The up-and-down stimulation needs to be continued for 15–45 seconds.

The choice of acupoints for migraine is best according to the painful site, which when well localized, would mean one to two points of puncture; or when unclearly localized and broad, could mean three to five points. Careful palpation is required to identify the most favourable sites of puncture. All those points are referred as Ashi points. For the frequent migraine sufferers, leaving the needles in for 20–30 min, with or without electrical stimulation, could be recommended. Patients need to be prepared for several rounds of treatment, each lasting about 10–20 days.

Occasionally, treating migraine with acupuncture could be associated with nausea and vomiting, which could be the accompanying symptoms of migraine or are induced by the acupuncture. With such knowledge or experience, local puncturing could be coupled with conventional punctures to prevent nausea and vomiting. Moreover, acupuncturists could also combine puncturing with herbal treatment when acupuncture alone fail to achieve desirable results.

References

Cui, S.M., Zhao, X.L., Zhao, M.L. (2005) Point injection treatment of 50 patients with angioneurotic headache. *Forum Tradit. Chin. Med.* **20**(3), 35.

Gu, W. Effect of Anshen acupoints acupuncture on angioneurotic headache. *Tianjin J. Tradit. Chin. Med.* **22**(3), 213–214.

Jia, C.S., Ma, X.S., Shi, J., *et al.* (2004) Acupuncture with electric stimulation at Qiuxu (GB 40) for migraine: A Multi-center randomized controlled clinical study. *J. Tradit. Chin. Med.* **8**(9), 814–817.

Li, A.Z. (1997) Effects of ear point taping and pressing therapy on T-lymphocyte subgroups in peripheral blood in children. *Chin. Acupunct. Moxibustion* **12**, 739.

Li, Y.C. and Ren, S.M. (1991) Clinical observation of point injection treatment of 105 patients with neurovascular headache. *Med. J. Chin. PLA* **16**(5), 331.

Liu, F.Y. and Xu, Y.X. (2003) Clinical observation of *Weizhong* and *Yanglingquan* acupoint injection with *Hong Dan injection* to treat 100 patients with migraine. *New J. Tradit. Chin. Med.* **35**(8), 54.

Liu, H. and Liu, H.L. (2002) Clinical observation on acupuncture treatment for 76 cases of nerve-vascular headache. *Chin. Acupunct. Moxibustion* **22**(5), 297–298.

Wang, X.Y. (2004) Clinical studies of the temperature acupuncture treatment of angioneurotic headache. *J. Guiyang Coll. Tradit. Chin. Med.* **26**(4), 33–35.

Wang, Z., Guo, Z.X. and Ma, W. (2002) Clinical observations on pricking blood treatment of migraine with three-edged needle. *Shanghai J. Acupunct. Moxibustion* **21**(3), 11–12.

Xing, J.Q. (1995) Efficacy analysis of acupuncture treatment of 108 patients with vascular headache. *Acta Academiae Medicinae Nanjing* **15**(4), 923.

Yang, L.F. and Xiao, Y.X. (2000) The plum-blossom needle treatment of 56 patients with migraine. *Shanxi. J. Tradit. Chin. Med.* **16**(5), 41.

Yu, W., Shen, M.X., Weng, Z.F., *et al.* (2000) Clinical research in acupuncture treatment of acute attack of vascular headache. *Shanghai J. Acupunct. Moxibustion* **19**(2), 15–16.

Yuan, J., Fang, J.Y., Li, M., *et al.* (2004) Clinical observation on migraine due to hemorheological abnormality in the treatment of acupuncture therapy according to TCM differentiation of syndromes. *Hebei J. Tradit. Chin. Med.* **26**(5), 361–363.

Zhang, J.P. and Qu, Z.Y. (1988) "Tapping Therapy" treatment of 35 patients with vascular headache. *J. Gansu Coll. Tradit. Chin. Med.* **2**, 30.

Zhu, G.X. and Chen, Z.G. (1999) Temperature acupuncture treatment of 62 patients with elderly intractable migraine. *Zhejiang J. Tradit. Chin. Med.* **5**, 212.

Chapter 8

Acupuncture for Stroke

Abstract

The clinical treatment of stroke includes the use of thrombolytic agents, followed by anticoagulation, control of intracranial pressure and blood pressure, possibly vascular surgery and related therapeutic measures. This chapter introduces an overview of the clinical applications of acupuncture and moxibustion on stroke during various stages.

Keywords: Stroke; Neurological Function; Convalescence.

8.1 Use of Acupuncture During the Acute Stage of Stroke

The treatment principles of stroke in the acute phase may include the following: improvement of the brain perfusion, reduction of nervous injury in the affected cerebral area, and control of cerebral edema.

The application of acupuncture in the acute phase of stroke is widely practised in China and has been supported by a great deal of clinical studies.

8.1.1 *Acute phase — immediately after stroke*

Hand Twelve Wells Points, viz. bulateral LU 11, LI 1, PC 9, TE 1, HT 9, SI 1, have been traditionally used for bloodletting using three-edged needle-pins immediately after occurrence of stroke. The classical teachings says that unconscious patients might wake up with such maneuvers.

(1) Fifty-two acute stroke patients (cerebral infarction and cerebral hemorrhage) in coma have been studied with bloodletting at the 12 points. Thirty cases received the meridian pricking and bloodletting

(16 with cerebral hemorrhage and 14 with cerebral infarction), and 22 cases were controls (13 with cerebral hemorrhage and 9 with cerebral infarction). The 12 acupoints were pricked with three-edged needles, and the amount of blood let out was one drop. Observations were made before pricking, and 15, 30 and 45 min after pricking for changes in their consciousness, blood pressure, breathing and pulse. The determination of consciousness was based on the Glasgow consciousness score. It was found that after meridian pricking and bloodletting on the hands, patients with small areas of cerebral injury became more conscious, systolic blood pressure rose, heart rate became faster, and there was not much influence on the respiration. For patients with medium areas of injury, the meridian pricking and bloodletting on the hand also improved their state of consciousness. However, those in the control group also improved, and no conclusion could be made. For patients with large areas of injury, no improvement was observed (Guo *et al.*, 2003).

(2) To observe the effects on the neurological function of patients suffering from acute stroke using acupuncture, 42 patients suffering from cerebral infarction within one week of attack were treated with Electro-Acupuncture (EA) (20 cases) or herbal medicine (22 cases) randomly. The medicine group used Danshen Root (Radix Salviae Miltiorrhizae), low molecular dextran and supporting treatment in accordance with the symptoms, and the EA group received standard treatment as well as EA. The acupoints selected and operation methods were as follows: GV 20, GV 24, LI 14, PC 6, LI 11, LR 3, SP 6 and ST 36. After filiform needles were inserted at those points, the twirling method was used in acuesthesia (feeling of local soreness, numbness, distention and heaviness), then G6805 EA treatment instrument was connected with dilatational wave, frequency at 5–45 Hz, and strength was within the patients' endurance limit, about 3 mA. Needles were retained for 30 min. EA was applied once daily, treatment was given for five days followed by a rest of two days, and the treatment course lasted for 5–7 weeks. An evaluation of patients' "extent of nervous functional disorder" was made in accordance with the "Confirmed Treatment Effect Standards, the Second National Cerebrovascular Disease Academic Conference". The results indicated

that there was significant recovery of the nervous functional disorder in the two groups of patients, and the recovery of the disorder in patients of the EA group was apparently better than that of the herbal medicine group. In addition, it was also observed that in terms of the recovery of the nervous functional disorder in patients treated with EA, the recovery of their muscle strength of the shoulder, hand and lower limb were more remarkable, and there was hardly any significant influence with regard to their consciousness and language.

(3) In another study trying to compare the effects of acupuncture together with thrombolytic treatment, 80 cases of acute cerebral infarction patients within 12 hours after the attack were randomly divided into acupuncture group and control group, each 40 cases. The control group was given acute phase stroke thrombolytic urokinase therapy, once daily. For the acupuncture group, in addition to urokinase, acupuncture was applied to the following selected acupoints: PC 6, GV 26, SP 6, GB 20, HT 1, LU 5, LI 4 and BL 40. Evaluation was made in accordance with the grading method of "Stroke diagnosis and evaluation standard (Trial)" (Encephalopathy Acute Collaborative Group of State Administration of Traditional Chinese Medicine, 1996) to evaluate patients' consciousness activities, language, limbs movement function and other symptomatic changes before and after treatment. Treatment effects were evaluated according to the following formula: (evaluation before treatment — evaluation after treatment) ÷ evaluation before treatment × 100%. On completion of the treatment course, more than 81% of the symptoms and adverse physical signs of both groups were reduced. The functional evaluation of the two groups of patient was conducted 30 days after treatment. The results of the data showed that there was no significant difference in the overall effective rate between the two groups. However, the improvement rate of acupuncture group was better than the medical treatment group. It was revealed therefore that application of acupuncture and thrombolytic in a combined treatment at the early phase could significantly increase therapeutic effects. The suggestion of synergism between the two treatments may have indicated the importance of early acupuncture intervention.

(4) Scalp needling is mainly used for neurological diseases, so it is widely applied in treating stroke. In the case of routine thrombolytic treatment on acute phase cerebral ischemia, scalp needling has been applied at the same time, and was reported to have better auxiliary effects. One study looked at 60 cases of cerebral ischemia within 12 hours of the stroke. They were divided randomly into the thrombolytic treatment group (30 cases) and the thrombolytic treatment plus scalp acupuncture group (30 cases). All patients met the following requirements: first time internal carotid artery thrombosis, suffered attack within 12 hours, excluded from brain hemorrhage by CT examination, no source of emboli, no accompanied infection, diabetes, and general complications, and a neurological evaluation score greater than 10 (Encephalopathy Acute Collaborative Group of State Administration of Traditional Chinese Medicine, 1996). The standard thrombolytic treatment included a total quantity of 60–75 thousand units of urokinase, followed by routine treatment. For the scalp acupuncture group, on top of the thrombolytic treatment, additional scalp acupuncture treatment was given. The acupuncture points selected were GV 20 to GB 7. The needles were retained for 8–12 hours, during which needle manipulation was done 2–4 times, each for 3–5 min. Acupuncture was done once daily, and the two groups were under observation for four weeks. Evaluation was based on neurological return assay with transcranial Doppler (TCD), detection of plasma t-PA (tissue plasminogen activator) activity, and concentration of plasma FG to observe the effect of treatment. The results indicated that the two groups of patients showed significant neurological improvement one hour after treatment and after four weeks, and the scalp acupuncture group at each point of time (one hour, one day, one week and four weeks after treatment) showed better improvement and better improved blood flow. Ten minutes after intromission of urokinase to scalp needling, patients' plasma t-Pa activity was immediately increased, and remained higher than those in the non-acupuncture group. The decline of plasma fibrinogen (FG) content of patients in the scalp acupuncture group was also significantly better than that of the control group. Judging from the results, it was suggested that scalp acupuncture took advantage of the "time

window" for reperfusion, and through the improvement of the brain circulation and increased blood flow, thereby protecting the ischemic area, the reperfusion injury was reduced to a minimum, and prevented further thrombosis.

(5) In another clinical report, it was found that the use of lesion localization encircled acupuncture gave better results than scalp acupuncture in treating acute phase cerebral ischemia. Sixty-one patients within a week of the acute attack of cerebral ischemia were divided randomly into encircled acupuncture group (31 cases) and scalp acupuncture group (30 cases). The encircled acupuncture was based on the computed tomography (CT) location of the lesion, taking the ipsilateral scalp projection area as the site to encircle, and using numbers 28–30 one-inch needles inserted at 30°. Pointing to the direction of the projection centre, each needle was inserted at intervals of 2 cm around the selected location. While needle was retained, manipulation of needle was carried out once every other 5 min. For the scalp acupuncture group, the hemiplegic contralateral motor area and sensation area were selected. The needle type, insertion angle and needling method were all the same as the encircling method. Both groups were matched with other acupuncture points in accordance with their syndrome differentiation that was due to imbalances of functions in liver, lung, or blood. Acupuncture was applied once daily for a treatment course of 30 days. The treatment evaluation was carried out in accordance with the 1996 formulated standard called "The Standard of Stroke Diagnosis and Treatment Evaluation". The results indicated that the treatment effect of encircled acupuncture group was significantly better than that of scalp acupuncture group. It was also found that both types of head acupuncture could lower the acute stroke patients' plasma content of arterenol and adrenaline, thereby cutting down the neurological damage and secondary brain injury due to abnormal release of arterenol and adrenaline.

Reports of application of acupuncture and moxibustion on acute phase of cerebral infarction are not limited to these; what have been recorded in different documents involving the use of acumoxi prescriptions may not be the same, yet the resulting observations provided all indicate that the early introduction of acumoxi in

the treatment of acute phase of cerebral infarction has positive significance. Such results are not only proven by clinical practices, they are
also supported by a large amount of clinical experimental research
findings.

(6) It was found that if EA was applied to GV 26, it could quickly
increase the cerebral blood flow of the ischemic hippocampus, and
subsequently reduced the injury of neurological tissues due to
ischemia. Acupuncture to PC 6 could significantly increase the blood
volume of the brain, affecting areas of low blood supply more
significantly (Yin and Shu, 1989)

After applying EA to ST 36 for 5 min, it was observed that there
was significant increase of blood flow in the microcirculation of the
brain, which was retained until 60 min after the needle was removed.
Scalp acupuncture could strengthen part of the cerebral blood flow
(Xiang *et al.*, 1996).

When scalp acupuncture was applied to rat, it could significantly
improve cerebral ischemia induced by cerebral arterial blocking through
lengthening of passive conditioned reflex latency, lowering of whole
blood viscosity, shrinking the cerebral infarction area, growing capillar-
ies in the necrotic lesion, and reducing edema and inflammation reactions of brain tissues surrounding the ischemia lesion.

(7) In the process of cerebral ischemia and reperfusion, the degeneration
and even death of neurons are closely related to the increased effect
of membrane lipid peroxidation, declining ability to clear free radicals
and abnormal energy metabolism. Acupuncture applied to acupoints
GV 20 and LI 11 could improve effectively delay injury to the nervous
due to ischemic reperfusion, effectively inhibit lipid peroxidation, and
raise the antioxidation ability.

After cerebral ischemia has occurred, there will be an accumulation
of Ca^{2+}, an overload of which will lead to serious brain injury.
Literatures suggested that there is no activity of Ca^{2+} itself, and its
activity is given the full effect when it combines with CaM to form
CA^{2+}-CaM compound (Yang, 1996). In animal experiments, it was
discovered that after cerebral ischemia, the content of cerebral active
CaM increases significantly, and applying acupuncture to GV 26 and
Well points could inhibit levels of active CaM in the brain cells.

Cerebral ischemia and reperfusion are obviously initiating complicated molecular changes at the cellular and molecular levels of the intracranial tissues. Scientific studies relying on molecular markers have repeated shown that EA induces remarkable changes in the biochemical markers related to cerebral regeneration. How does EA affect such changes still remains speculative.

8.2 Use of Acupuncture for Stroke Convalescence

Stroke convalescence starts two weeks after the cerebral vascular accident, stretching to one to six months after. After stabilization from the acute phase, stroke patients might have remaining symptoms, like selective paralysis or paresis, language difficulties, dysphagy, incontinence, etc.

8.2.1 *Acupuncture for hemiplegia after stroke*

Paralysis is the most common outcome of cerebrovascular accident. The clinical presentation of neurological defect depends on the severity of injury and speed of restoration. Paralysis induced by stroke can be divided into two types. One type is induced by the injury of pyramidal cells or pyramidal tract, which is also called upper motorneuron paralysis or central paralysis, whose characteristics are reflected in patients' rigidity and hypertonicity; another type is induced by the injury of cerebral neuromotor nucleus and its tissues, which is also called lower motorneuron paralysis or peripheral paralysis, whose characteristic is embodied in member's flaccid paralysis, weakness and lack of strength (Chen and Zhou, 2001). The recovery process after stroke hemiplegia, according to Brunnstrom, could be divided into six stages, viz. (1) atony (no reflex) stage; (2) mild spasms, may be combined with reactions; (3) aggravated spasms, could voluntarily induce chained reactions; (4) weakened spasms, with dissociative motion; (5) established autonomous motion; and (6) motion approaching normal. For simplicity, we could consider two periods viz. Period of flaccid paralysis and Spastic Period, in subsequent discussions.

8.2.2 *Period of flaccid paralysis*

The characteristics of flaccid paralysis period are manifested in the reduction of muscle tension, weakening or disappearance of tendon reflex, and absence of pathological reflex. Clinically the affected side appears to be in flaccid paralysis with total loss of strength. The "flaccid paralysis period" is due to the loss of control of motion by the higher neurological centers so that the affected side becomes flaccid. The principle of this early period of restoration treatment on hemiplegia should be on the raising of muscle tension to shorten the soft paralysis period so that the spastic stage can be entered earlier than normal. Chinese Medicine maintains that "the brain is the house of spirit light", and during the "flaccid paralysis period", as the brain is invaded by all evils, the orifice is clouded, giving rise to malfunction of spirit, causing the loss of control of the meridians, and as a result muscles become flaccid. The principle of treatment should be arousing the spirit and purging the excessiveness, and freeing the channels and networks. Clinical studies showed that during the soft paralysis period, applying acupuncture excites the peripheral nerves and thus the recovery of the paralyzed muscles could be promoted.

According to the Brunnstrom's hemiplegia recovery theory, the upper limb flexors would be first restored, followed by the lower limb extensors. The major trouble in the "flaccid paralysis period" is the attenuation or loss of muscle tension, and treatment should use facilitative method to promote the production and strengthening of the muscle tension. At this time using acupuncture to stimulate agonistic muscles as an afferent of peripheral feeling, to excite γ motor neurons, facilitating lower centre of spinal chord in reflexive induction in producing and increasing muscle tension would be appropriate. At the same time, α motor neurons could also be excited to promote the generation of dissociated motion, facilitating recovery of muscle strength of the paralyzed muscles. Along the four limbs, most of the flexor-related acupuncture points are on the paths of the Yin Meridians whereas the extensors are on the Yang Meridians. The so-called installment of balanced acupuncture is based on this fact to work out the acupoints prescription. In one study on of post-stroke soft paralyzed patients within one week of the stroke, 100 cases were randomly divided into two groups of 50 cases. The acupuncture points selected for treatment were as follows: for those suffering from lateral upper limbs, Yin Meridian points were selected; for lower limbs, Yang Meridian points were selected; and for the control group, upper and lower limbs Yang Meridian points were selected. EA — with frequencies of 10–100 Hz, disperse and dense waves, and stimulation within patients' maximum endurance — was applied for half an hour. A treatment course comprises six days; then after one day's rest, the next treatment course was given. After two weeks of treatment, patients' muscle tension in the treatment group was transformed from grade 0 to grade 1, and most of them could achieve satisfactory results within eight weeks without going through the spastic phase. After treatment for 60 days, a recovery evaluation test was made, in which the accumulated score of the treatment group patients was found higher than those of the control group, in terms of time required to reach grade 1 muscle tension, lowering muscle spasm and enhancing motor function.

There is a record on the understanding of the pathomechanism of stroke hemiplegia in *"Ling Shu"*, an ancient Chinese Medicine Classic, which instructed that to restore the damaged *qi*, "contralateral meridian needling method should be adopted, i.e. to treat left side take the right, and to treat the right side, to be the left". This means; when the left side is paralyzed, apply acupuncture treatment on the right side, and vice versa.

To compare the clinical effects of acupuncture points selected from the affected side, a study was conducted on 114 cases of post-stroke patients. They were randomly divided into research observation group A and treatment control group B. The A Group had 65 patients, and B group had 49. Treatment for A Group — Brunnstrom Stage I and II patients — was acupuncture on the healthy side: LU 10, L 14, SJ 5, LI 13 and LI 15 with strong stimulating needling, twice daily, with the needle retained for 15 min every time. On the morbid side, LU 10 was selected, using stronger stimulating needling but without retaining the needle, twice daily. Treatment for B group was acupuncture on the morbid side for LU 10, LI 4, TE 5, LI 11, LI 10, LI 15 and ST 11 once daily, and the needle was retained for 30 min every time. The results showed that after treatment, the A Group patients' upper limb function recovered rapidly, and upon discharge from hospital, their upper limb function and daily activity were significantly better those of B Group. This observation could be a modern demonstration of the merits of the classical teaching. According to modern neurophysiological principles, when the muscle with stronger strength contracts voluntarily, all motor neurons are gathered in excitement, thus reinforcing the muscle of weaker strength and promoting the beginning of the recovering process of the weaker muscles. After a treatment course of three months, 61.54% of A Group patients reached early stage of recovery, whereas only 38.78% of B Group did as well. The author also reminded us that once the patients showed the increase of muscle tension, further provocation should be stopped, lest the upper limb might go into the spastic phase by mistake.

8.2.3 *Spastic period*

As a stroke patient enters the spastic period, due to lower nerve centre taking over the overall activities, the unopposed release of motor activity induces the muscle tension to a morbid level, resulting in spasms, tendon reflex accentuation and pathological reflexes. The patient's tight upper limb flexor spasms, simultaneous with the lower limb's full extension spasms, are characteristics of the hemiplegia. With the development of this condition, the aggravation of the spasms is reflected mainly as involuntary movement of associated reaction and concomitant movements. When the spasms are under control, the associated abnormal movements will gradually settle before active, voluntary isolated movements will re-appear and limb function restored.

In Classical Chinese Medicine theory, post-stroke hemiplegia is the result of "liver wind" causing internal disturbances. Clinically, these theories have direct guiding effects on acupuncture prescriptions.

Both the channel sinew and *yang ming* schools of acupuncture have been used as treatment methods.

(1) Forty-eight cases of hospitalized patients suffering from post-stroke hemiplegia were studied. They were divided according to random numbers into channel sinew needling group (24 cases) and *yang ming* needling group. The acupoints selected in channel sinew needling group were based on the tender spots found by pressing along the medial and lateral sides of tendons and ligaments around the joints such as shoulder, elbow, wrist, fingers, knee and ankles of the patient. The points selected were ST 8, GB 4, CV 17, CV 16, SI 18, ST 3 and CV 1. For the *yang ming* group the points selected were LI 15, LI 11, LI 10, TE 5, LI 4, ST 31, ST 34, ST 36, ST 41 and SP 6. Acupuncture needles were retained for 30 min, and manipulated every

other 5–7 min. Needling was applied once daily, 30 sessions forming a course, for a total of three courses. Using Brunnstrom's six stage method to evaluate the grade changes before and after treatment, SIAS method to evaluate stroke patient's overall functional conditions, Ashworth method to evaluate spasm state, and using self-designed isodynamic time quantitative measuring method to evaluate the conditions of muscle (function), the results suggested that the channel sinew needling was significantly better than *yang ming* method in terms of spasm relief and improvement of joint movements. A further study revealed that both methods could significantly lower the pressure of patients' cerebrospinal fluid, Glu/GABA ratio, and increase the content of GABA but channel sinew needling group was better than *yang ming* needling group.

According to modern rehabilitation theory for the treatment of spastic paralysis, the emphasis should be put on the balance of coordination between muscle groups. Attention should be paid on the strengthening of upper limb extensor and lower limb flexor movements, coordinating and balancing the muscle tension of agonistic muscle and antagonistic muscle, enhancing concomitant movements towards transformation of dissociative movements, inhibiting and controlling spasms, and establishing normal mode of movement. In accordance with these principles, respective acupoints were selected from the upper limb flexor group, HT 1, LU 6, PC 7; the extensor group, LI 15, TE 10, TE 4; the lower limb extensor group, BL 36, SP 10, KI 6; and the flexor group, ST 31, LR 8, BL 62. Needling was first applied to the better side, with heavier lifting and thrusting manipulations. Then needling continued on the worse side, with light and soft twirling and turning manipulations, which is called "balanced tension needling". The traditional needling group selected the following acupoints: LI 15, LI 11, TE 5, LI 4, GB 34, GB 30, LR 3, GB 38, BL 60 and ST 36. The results showed that balanced tension needling achieved an effective rate of 93.75% in relieving lateral muscle tension and this was significantly much more effective than the traditional needling group (effective rate, 83.33%).

(2) Two hundred cases of patients with hemiplegia after stroke were randomly divided into four groups of 50 each. Group A received

acupuncture and facilitation, Group B just facilitation, Group C just acupuncture and Group D received routing drug treatment. For the acupuncture group, EA was applied on acupoints selected from the hand and foot *yang ming* meridians of the morbid side. For those hemiplegic patients in the late stages, additional acupunctures according to the general "pattern differentiation" could be added. Acupuncture was done once daily, with the needle retained for 20–30 min. For facilitation, the Bobath technique was mainly used for training which was given once daily, each time lasting 30–40 min. The results of the study showed that Groups A, B, C enjoyed better improvement of spasms than Group D. The results for Group B patients after treatment in the late stages were no different from those of Group C, while Group A patients did much better than Groups B and C. Results suggested that acupuncture coupled with facilitation could promote the restoration of functional movements of the stroke patient with hemiplegia.

8.2.4 *Acupuncture for the treatment of dysphagia after stroke*

Dysphagia after stroke is mostly due to unilateral or bilateral corticopontine tract injury, affecting the ambiguous nucleus of the muscle groups controlling throat movements and the nucleus of the hypoglossal nerve which controls tongue movements. More serious symptoms occurred if the medulla oblongata is also damaged. Dysphagia present with difficulties in soft palate, throat, and tongue movements. Swallowing, articulation and talking are affected, but the pharyngeal reflex is unaffected while mandibular reflex is strengthened. To compensate for the defects, nose or gastrostomy feeding might be necessary to maintain nutritional needs, thus seriously affecting the quality of life.

The incidence of dysphagia after stroke is about 45%, for which 86% will recover within 14 days after the attack (*Gordon et al.*, 1987). For the treatment of persistent dysphagia, there is yet hardly any standard effective method. Acupuncture is a practical consideration.

(1) To study the treatment effect of acupuncture on dysphagia after stroke, a study was conducted in which 90 cases of conscious patients

with over 30 days of dysphagia were randomly divided into an acupuncture group of 60 cases, and a rehabilitation training group of 30 cases. Acupoints selected included GV 16, ST 9, CV 23 and GV 14. At GV 16, a 2 cm filiform needle was used with its tip pointing towards the Adam's apple to penetrate 1.2 cm, until the feeling of acuasthenia. At ST 9, 1.5 cm lateral to the Adam's apple and medial to the common carotid artery, a 2 cm needle was inserted for 1.8 cm. At CV 23, a 3 cm filiform needle was used and at GV 14, a 2 cm filiform needle, where perpendicular penetrations were made. For the rehabilitation training group, procedures were carried out according to Logemann's training recommendations, and evaluation of results was based on the swallowing function. The acupuncture group achieved a cure rate of 31.7%, effectiveness rate of 61.6% and a total effectiveness rate 93.3%, which was better than that of the control group. Further observations revealed that acupuncture treatment did better with cerebropontine damages than bulbar palsy.

(2) Another study on 30 stroke patients with dysphagia looked at the electromyogram of the swallowing muscles 5 min before and after treatment, as well as the brain stem evoked potential. It was found that true bulbar palsy patients enjoyed normal crircothyroid muscle, and tongue muscle electromyogram after acupuncture. For cerebropontine damage, there was no significant change in the electromyograms before and after needling, although treatment effect seemed to be significant.

(3) Classical recommendations for the acupuncture treatment of dysphagia do exist. These include "Jin's 3 needles" (Chen and Jin, 2006) to improve speech disorder, throat irritation and dysphagia. The "3 brain needles" are GV 17 and bilateral GB 19. The "3 tongue needles" are *Shàng Lián Quán* (EX-HN20) and the two acupoints 0.8 cm to the left and right of it. Scalp needling (Zhang, 2005) and body needling are usually used in combination to strengthen treatment effect.

8.2.5 *Acupuncture for the treatment of language difficulty after stroke*

Language disorder is a common symptom after stroke. Cerebral hemorrhage, infarction and ischemia could all lead to aphasia. The occurrence and extent of aphasia are mainly related to the damage to the language centre. With the widespread application of CT and MRI on the brain, more and more observations revealed that apart from the "language center", damage of some cortical areas and deep structures could also lead to aphasia (Zhu *et al.*, 1998).

Although natural recovery is expected, the extent depends on the nature and size of the lesion. Speech therapists have a hard tissue rehabilitating the affected. Acupuncture treatment could be tried.

(1) One study on the acupuncture treatment effect of aphasia after stroke, recruited 88 patients with post-stroke aphasia. They were randomly divided into an acupuncture group of 30 cases, a scalp needling group of 30 cases and language rehabilitation training group of 28 cases. For the acupuncture group, the following acupoints were selected: GV 20, GB 7, HT 5, KI 6, together with pricking on the tongue surface. Needles were retained for two hours before withdrawal. The tongue surface was divided into nine areas based on front, middle and back with middle and right regions. All nine areas were pricked with a superfine needle at a fast speed. Slight bleeding (about 2 ml) was allowed. For the scalp acupuncture group, acupoints were selected on the focus side of the language 1 area (left). All three groups received treatment once daily, six times as one treatment course, with a total of four treatment courses. The results indicated that the acupuncture group had an effectiveness rate of 93.33%, traditional scalp needling group, 76.66%, while language rehabilitation group, 64.28%. After comparing the effects before and after treatment, it was found that all three methods had significant treatment effects, but the acupuncture treatment group did best, scalp needling group second, and language rehabilitation group third.

(2) The tongue stimulating method is becoming popular in the treatment of language disorder after stroke. The selection of acupoints may vary, but the aim is to locally stimulate the tongue. For example the "tongue 3-points" method (Lai, 1997) puts the first puncture to CV 23, and the second and third needle are applied 1 cm to the left and right. Needles are retained for 20–30 min with intermittent manipulations.

(3) Another study using CT imaging to determine the focus of treatment and applying acupuncture around the periphery of the vertical

projection of the lesion on the ipsilateral scalp had been completed. Four to eight 1.5 cm filiform needles were used to encircle the lesion with the puncture directions all pointing towards the centre of the image area. When there was acuesthesia felt, the acupuncturist would use a frequency rate of 180–200 time/min to twirl and turn for 2 min, and the needles were retained for 30 min. In addition, acupuncture using other acupoints, GV 15, CV 23 and HT 5, could be used simultaneously. Results showed that the treatment effect was significantly better than traditional scalp acupuncture.

8.2.6 *Acupuncture treatment for hand swelling after stroke*

After a stroke, the affected upper limb commonly suffers from swelling, pain and loss of mobility, known as shoulder-hand syndrome. A study was conducted on 26 patients suffering from this syndrome after stroke, and 20 other cases of stroke patients not suffering from shoulder-hand syndrome. EA treatment was given to the former group. The acupoints selected were on the morbid side, HT 1, LI 15, PC 3, LI 11, TE 5, PC 6, TE 4, PC 7, LI 4 and PC 8. Needling was given once daily with 14 days as a treatment course, then resting for two days before repeating, giving a total of three treatment courses. The results indicated that patients suffering from shoulder-hand syndrome enjoyed better microcirculation when compared with the control group, when their nail beds were examined for the state of blood flow, red cells gathering and exudation bleeding etc. It was also found that acupuncture gave better results. This suggested that EA improved shoulder-hand syndrome through improving patient's microcirculation disorder (Xia, 1998).

8.3 The Application of Acupuncture Treatment in the Late Period after Stroke

During the late stage after stroke patients often suffer from muscles atrophy, and continual deterioration. The use of acupuncture might have special indications. Muscles atrophy after stroke could have been caused by the deprivation of nutrients to vascular networks and treatment could rely on the traditional belief of spleen-fortification and *qi*-boosting, and circulation promotion using the following acupoints: SP 10, ST 36, SP 6 and CV 6. For facial muscle atrophy, the following could be added: BL 2, EX-HN 4 and ST 2. For swallowing difficulty, the following could be added: GB 20, GV 15, CV 22 and CV 23. For inability to raise the head, the following could be added: BL 10 and GB 20. For strengthening the four limbs, the following could be added: LI 15, LI 11, TE 5, LI 4, GB 30, GB 34 and LR. According to the theory of "treating atrophy only take the *yang ming* meridian" (as *yang ming* meridians are full of *qi* and blood), acupoints from the hand-foot *yang ming* meridians are particularly suitable for muscle atrophy.

In modern physiotherapy, the low frequency pulse electrical treatment method, such as neuromy-electrostimulation therapy (or functional electrostimulation, FES), is often used to prevent muscle atrophy. It stimulates denervated muscles, leading to their rhythmic contractions, promoting local blood flow which improves tissue metabolism, promotes regeneration of nerve fibers and restores the transmission function. The EA therapy used in acupuncture treatment is exactly this type of low frequency pulse current, to restore muscle contractions.

8.3.1 *Influence of acupuncture on the arterial state of stroke patients*

ET is a vascular endothelial peptide which has a strong vasoconstriction effect. It has three types: ET-1, ET-2 and ET-3, of which the vasoconstriction activity of ET-1 is the strongest (Volpe and Cosentino, 2000.). Function disorders of ET is one of the common factors causing a series of pathological changes leading to stroke. After ET is released from endothelial cells, it first combines with a ET receptor on the surface of the target cell, leading to many kinds of membrane reactions, aggravating cerebral tissues damages (Cosentino *et al.*, 2001). A clinical study was conducted on patients suffering from transient ischemic attack where there was insufficient cerebral blood supply. An increase of plasma ET level was revealed in both cerebral infarction and transient ischemic patients, but the level was much higher in the former. It was also found that the larger the area of cerebral infarction, the more significant the increase of the plasma ET level which did not fall (Xu *et al.,* 1995).

Scalp needling on healthy subjects has been found to significantly reduce the content of plasma endothelial peptides in stroke patient

(Zhang *et al.*, 2006). It was found that puncturing GV 20, HT 5, SP 6, and coupled with EA, significantly lowered the level of ET in patient's plasma. The effect was even better than using cerebrolysin 20 ml in an intravenous drip, together with nimodipine, and aspirin. With regard to studies on stroke patients with carotid arthroma, puncturing PC 6, GB 20, ST 40 and ST 36, significantly lowers patients' blood ET levels and increases CGRP levels (Wang *et al.*, 2005).

8.4 Other Observations

The popularity in using acupuncture at different stages of stroke and the many interesting beneficial effects observed have led to further clinical and experimental research on the influence of acupuncture on the specific areas of cellular and molecular changes during the different stages of stroke. These specific areas includes:

(1) Hemorrheology, where changes in blood viscosity, blood volume, cellular compositions and biochemical indices etc., have been found to be affected by acupuncture.

(2) Oxygen free radical releases, where the free radicals contribute towards the further development of atheroma. Acupuncture has been observed to suppress the releases significantly.

(3) Cellular and molecular changes are manifested in the electrical picture of cerebral activities, viz. EEG. The recent utilization of MRI has revealed a lot of functional activities initiated by acupuncture. Before MRI, EEG changes have long been observed to change with acupuncture of different intentions.

8.5 Summary

In recent years, there has been extensive interest on the use of acupuncture for the treatment of stroke. Clinical and experimental studies are plentiful. During the acute phase, an early administration of acupuncture treatment achieved better auxiliary treatment effects, and is conducive to better recovery in the rehabilitation period. During the rehabilitation period, a combination of modern rehabilitative technology together with acupuncture treatment could further improve the clinical achievements.

Even during the very late stage when modern medicine has nothing to offer, acupuncture remains a viable option.

Clinical studie on the application of acupuncture in the various phases of stroke are plentiful. However, with regard to animal experiments, almost all experimental studies focused on the acute phase and late results are lacking.

To date, rescue measures for acute stroke are basically perfect, enabling most patients to safely pass over to the restoration period for rehabilitative treatment. The final stroke sequel, however, remains a serious problem for all patients. Although the present treatment effect of acupuncture on the stroke sequel is yet short of standardized procedures, not to speak of guaranteed results, acupuncture is a valuable offer to many patients.

On the experimental side, the new Middle Cerebral Artery Occlusion (MCAO) model would lead to new series of studies on different treatment modalities including acupunctures.

Stroke is common. The survival rate after stroke is improving all the time with better resuscitations, better means of controlling hypertension and maintenance of cardiovascular health. Those who suffer from stroke, however, are frequently suffering from residual problems of neurological deficiencies, ranging from hemiplegia, hemiparesis, stiffness, spasm, speech problems and swallowing difficulties.

Conventional rehabilitation like different forms of physiotherapy do work, but often fail to achieve satisfactory results. Ever since the practice of acupuncture is maintained in China, it has been popularly used as a means to promote recovery for stroke patients. As acupuncture is becoming acceptable outside China, and ever since pain treatment using acupuncture is endorsed as a practical methodology, the application of acupuncture in post-stroke rehabilitation is becoming more and more popular. Special divisions in hospital rehabilitation units are organized, using acupuncture as standard means for neurological stimulations. Physical therapists and clinicians take special courses to learn the technique, and clinical research of various scales is conducted to explore the clinical evidences on its efficacy.

Acupuncture can cause multiple biological responses, including circulatory and biochemical effects. These responses can occur locally or close to the site of application, or at a distance. They are mediated mainly by sensory neurons to many structures within the central nervous system.

This can lead to activation of pathways affecting various physiological systems in the brain as well as in the periphery.

Acupuncture has been well accepted by Chinese patients and is widely used to improve motor, sensation, speech, and other neurological functions in patients with stroke. As a therapeutic intervention, acupuncture is also increasingly practiced in some Western countries. However, it remains uncertain whether the existing evidence is scientifically rigorous enough so that acupuncture can be recommended for routine use. However, we need to assess the efficacy and safety of acupuncture for patients with stroke in the subacute or chronic stage. A careful review of publications on the subject was done in 2006 (Wu *et al.*, 2009).

A sensitive electronic search of multiple reference databases was done in late 2005, including Cochrane Stroke Group Trials Registry, the Cochrane Complementary Medicine Field Trials Register, the Cochrane Central Register of Controlled Trials, MEDLINE (Ovid), EMBASE, CINAHL, AMED, the Chinese Biological Medicine Database, the National Center for Complementary and Alternative Medicine Register, and the National Institute of Health Clinical Trials Database. We included all randomized clinical trials among patients with ischemic or hemorrhagic stroke, in the subacute or chronic stage, which compared acupuncture involving needling with either placebo acupuncture, sham acupuncture, or no acupuncture. Two review authors independently selected trials for inclusion, assessed quality, extracted, and cross-checked the data.

Five trials (368 patients) met the inclusion criteria. Methodological quality was considered inadequate in all trials. Although the overall estimate from four trials suggested the odds of improvement in global neurological deficit was higher in the acupuncture group compared with the control group (odds ratio (OR) 6.55, 95% confidence interval (CI) 1.89–22.76), this estimate may not be reliable because there was substantial heterogeneity ($I^2 = 68\%$). One trial showed no significant improvement of motor function between the real acupuncture group and the sham acupuncture group (OR 9.00, 95% CI 0.40–203.30), but the confidence interval was wide and included clinically significant effects in both directions. No data on death, dependency, institutional care, change of neurological deficit score, quality of life, or adverse events were available.

This systematic review does not provide evidence to support the routine use of acupuncture for patients with subacute or chronic stroke.

The widespread use of acupuncture, the promising results with less severe side effects, lower cost, and the insufficient quality of the available trials warrant further research. Large sham or placebo-controlled trials are needed to confirm or refute the available evidence (Wu *et al.*, 2008).

Looking at the situation in China, using acupuncture as a tool for post-stroke recovery is taken as a common sense, accepted by patients and clinicians, clinics and hospitals. All forms and modalities of acupuncture are being used while the specific situations for indications are yet to be identified. Research is seldom conducted.

8.5.1 *Timing of application*

When stroke happens, there is a period of uncertainty: from survival to the period of loss of consciousness. Hence, most clinicians would not start acupuncture during the initial period. While most acupuncture practices start after the regain of full consciousness, some trials on earlier applications have commenced. Results are yet to be revealed on whether such energetic application would facilitate conscious recovery, better cognitive return or more favourable potential of neuromuscular rehabilitation. As patients demand better results, and clinicians are getting more ambitions, starting acupuncture at the very early stage o the stroke event should deserve serious explorations.

8.5.2 *Techniques and methodology*

Great varieties of treatment modalities have been applied in China, ranging from classical punctures, electrical acupunctures, ear punctures, acupoint injections, acupoint thread implants, moxibustion and hot vacuum cupping, etc. Acupuncturists have not worked out the indications, other than a free practice and individual adjustments according to their clinical judgment.

Basing on a fundamental understanding of neurology, the emphasis should be put on the stimulation of the affected side by promoting neurological recovery or mobilizing unaffected, undamaged components to take over or contribute towards the lost function. If the aim of the acupuncture is on muscle recovery, perhaps electrical enhancement of the acupuncture effect could be an important consideration.

The choice of acupuncture points needs more careful definitions. However, it has been widely accepted that during the flaccid stage, the acpoints along the Yin Meridian are used for the upper limb, while for the lower limb, those on the Yang Meridian are used. During the rigid stage, the reverse logic is applied. During the very late stage of rehabilitation, the choice of acupuncture points could follow the indications for treatment musculoskeletal problems.

8.5.3 *Difficult situations*

Stroke is often complicated with swallowing difficulties, phonation problems and limb oedema. The unpredictability of how spastic stiffness will develop is another problem affecting an intelligent choice of acupuncture points when treatment starts.

For swallowing difficulties, the usual choice is a collection of points relevant to tongue and throat function, like *Lian-quan* (CV23), *Jin-jin* (EX-HN12), *Yu-ye* (EX-HN13) and *Ren-ying* (ST9). Needling depth is recommended to be around 2 cm, aiming at the initiation of intense feeling of discomfort and choking sensation. It is not recommended that needles be left in place after the unusual stimulations.

For phonation problems, the acupoints and recommended procedures follow closely those of swallowing difficulties.

For limb oedema, when the affected limbs give a distal presentation, puncturing with bloodletting is recommended. The acupoints recommended include *Shi-xuan* (EX-UE11), *Ba-feng* (X-LE10), *Ba-xie* (EX-UE9) and *Si-feng* (EX-UE10).

References

Chen, J.P. and Zhou, G.D. (2001) *Integrative Medicine for the Treatment of Brain Vascular Diseases*. Peoples' Military Medical Press, Beijing, pp. 384–386.

Chen, X.H. and Jin, R. (2006) A clinical observation on treatment of apoplectic pseudobnlbar paralysis by Jin's three-needle manipulation. *New J. Tradit. Chin. Med.* **38**(7), 65–66.

Cosentino, F., Rubattu, S., Savoia, C., *et al.* (2001) Endothelial dysfunction and stroke. *J Cardiovasc. Pharmacol.* **38**(Suppl 2), S75–8.

Encephalopathy Acute Collaborative Group of State Administration of Traditional Chinese Medicine. (1996) Stroke diagnosis and evaluation standard (Trial). *J. Beijing Univ. Tradit. Chin. Med.* **19**(1), 55–56.

Gordon, C., Hewer, R.L. and Wade, D.T. (1987) Dysphagia in acute stroke. *Brit. Med. J.* **295**(15), 411–414.

Guo, Y., Wang, X., Xu, T., *et al.* (2003) Clinical observation of the influence of puncture and blood letting at twelve hand jing point on consciousness and heart rate in patients with wind-stroke. *Tianjin J. Tradit. Chin. Med.* **20**(2), 35–37.

Lai, X.S. (1997) Clinical application of tongue acupuncture for treatment of the language barrier. *J. Clin. Acupunct. Moxibustion* **13**(4,5), 17.

Volpe, M. and Cosentino, F. (2000) Abnormalities of endothelial function in the pathogenesis of stroke: The importance of endothelin. *J. Cardiovasc. Pharmacol.* **35**(4 Suppl 2), S45–48.

Wang, W., Wang Z. and Zhao J. (2005) Influence of acupuncture and moxibustion on lipid, blood flow deformation, LPO, SOD, ET and CGRP in patients with carotid atherosclerosis due to ischemic cerebrovascular diseases. *Shanghai J. Acupunct. Moxibustion* **24**(7), 19–23.

Wu, H., Tang, J., Lin, X., Lau, J., Leung, P.C., Woo, J. and Li, Y. (2009) Acupuncture for stoke rehabilitation (review). *Cochrane Library* (1): CD004131.

Xia, C. (1998) Effect about Changes of nailfold microcirculation with acupuncture in apoplectie hemiplegia with shoulder hand syndrome. *Chin. J. Microcirc.* **8**(2), 38–39.

Xiang, L., Wang H. and Li Z. (1996) TCD observation on cerebral blood flow dynamics inference of cerebral atrophy with scalp therapy. *Acupunct. Res.* **4**, 7–9.

Xu, X.R., Xing, Z.H., Yang, Y.D., *et al.* (1995) Dynamic change of plasma endothelin and its relations with the condition of stroke patients. *Chin. J. Nerv. Ment. Dis.* **21**(4), 219–222.

Yang, G. (1996) *Endocrine Physiology and Pathophysiology.* Tianjin Sci. Tech. Press, Tianjin, pp. 59–67.

Yin, J.H. and Shu, D.G. (1989) Observation of the brain impedance rheogram change before and after acupuncture at Neiguan. *Shandong Med. J.* **29**(3), 48–49.

Zhang, H.-X., Zhou, L. and Zhang T.-F. (2006) Effects of scalp acupuncture on related blood biochemical indexes in treatment of apoplexy. *Chin. J. Chin. Rehabil.* **10**(19): 9–12.

Zhang, Y. (2005) Clinical study of scalp acupuncture with body acupuncture treatment of pseudobulbar paralysis. *Study J. Tradit. Chin. Med.* **23**(5), 1129.

Zhu, C.H., Chen, W.X. and Li, H.J. (1998) The study of the relationship between speech disorders caused by acute cerebrovascular disease and the sites of lesions. *J. Clin. Neurol.* **11**(4), 234–235.`

Chapter 9

Acupuncture for Asthma

Abstract

Bronchial asthma is a common, respiratory disease related to allergy. The clinical symptoms include: break-out of dry cough, mostly accompanied with breathing difficulties, and a wheezing sound in exhalation. The etiology of asthma is complicated and it is often taken as a multigenic hereditary disease, affected by genetic and environmental factors. As the pathogenesis of asthma is complicated, the number of ways with which asthma is treated might not achieve satisfactory results. Acupuncture is good alternative treatment. Acupuncture might influence the autonomic system directly or might work through a series of humoral modulations which help to control inflammation and bronchial spasm.

Keywords: Asthma; Allergy; Moxibustion; Respiratory Function.

9.1 Treating Asthma with Acupuncture

To observe the therapeutic effects of acupuncture on asthma during its acute attack, a comparative group taking anti-asthmatics was studied. The acupoints selected were: *Zhigou* (支沟 SJ TE6), *Neiguan* (内关 PC6), *Taichong* (太冲 LR3), *Feishu* (肺俞 BL13), *Fenglong* (丰隆 ST40) and *Yinglingquan* (阴陵泉 SP9). The medication used in the comparative group was an anti-asthmatic vaporizer. The results did not show any marked difference between the effects of the two different groups (90% vs. 90%). When lung function tests were conducted on the patients, it was discovered that the influence of acupuncture on the lung function indices, such as forced vital capacity (FVC), the second forced expiratory volume in 1.0 s (FEV1.0) and peak expiratory flow rate (PEFR), were better than those from the medication group. The effects of acupuncture in lowering patients' interleukin-4 (IL-4) levels and increasing the interferon-gamma (IFN-γ) levels also surpassed that of the medication group. The T helper (Th1) cells, which mainly generate IFN-γ, could inhibit the production of IL-4 and counteract against its effect on the target cell. The Th2 cell mainly generated IL-4, promoted the integration of IgE, enhanced immunoresponse, and activated macrophage and mast cells, releasing imflammatory media, which suggested that acupuncture could be adjusting the imbalanced function between the Th1/Th2 subgroups to lower the inflammation and allergic reactions at the trachea, achieving a better result than clinical medication (Zhang *et al.*, 2005).

Bronchial asthma is a respiratory tract disease with early symptoms of reversible bronchial spasm exhaling difficulties, manifesting as panting. Applying acupuncture to *Yuji* (鱼际 LU10), *Zusanli* (足三里 ST35), *Guanyuan* (关元 RN CV4) and *Daizhui* (大椎 DU GV14) could markedly increase the lung's maximum ventilation capacity, vital capacity, FEV1.0 and deep exhaling capacity. It was found in a clinical study that treating *Yuji* (鱼际 LU10) with acupuncture could relieve or even eliminate the wheezing sound. It was inferred that the *Yuji* (鱼际 LU10) point could have the function of relieving bronchial spasm (Feng *et al.*, 1983).

Physiologically, the cyclic adenosine monophosphate (cAMP) and cyclic guanosine monophosphate (cGMP) are a pair of regulating factors, closely related to nitrogen containing hormonal effects. The levels of cAMP and cGMP in cells, particularly the cAMP/cGMP ratio, has an important effect on the tension of bronchial smooth muscles. As the second messenger, cAMP has the effect on the stabilization of bronchial smooth muscle membrane potential, expanding bronchiales, and preventing the attack of asthma. The cGMP in cells can accelerate the release of bioactivated material, stimulate the vagal receptors under the mucous membrane, initiate the constriction of bronchial muscles, and lead to the onset of asthma.

It was discovered that during the onset of asthma, patients' level of cAMP in plasma, the cAMP/cGMP ratio and the level of cortisol in plasma were lowered, while the level of cGMP was higher than those of normal people. Immediately and two weeks after applying acupuncture therapy to patients (with *Yuji* (鱼际 LU10) as major point of selection, supplemented by *Guanyuan* (关元 RN CV4), *Qihai* (气海 RN CV6) and *Daizhui* (大椎

DU GV14)), it was found that with the relief of wheezing and improvement of the symptoms, most patients' cAMP levels in plasma, cAMP/cGMP ratio, and the levels of cortisol in plasma, were significantly higher. On the other hand, the levels of cGMP in plasma became lowered. There was no such effect in normal people under the same effects of acupuncture. It was therefore inferred that acupuncture therapy of bronchial asthma could be related to the following mechanism: through acupuncture, patients' excitability of their sympathetic nerve became raised, and at the same time, the hyperfunction of their parasympathetic nerve became suppressed. This promoted the adrenal cortex function, increasing the level of cAMP and lowering the level of cGMP in their plasma and cells, and elevating the cAMP/cGMP ratio, which in turn reduces bronchial spasm and improves lung ventilation, leading to the relief of asthma (Feng *et al.*, 1983) .

9.2 Treating Asthma with Natural Moxibustion

Natural moxibustion is a kind of acupoint dressing therapy, also known as cold moxibustion, which uses stimulating medicinal herbs as dressings on specified acupoint's on the skin surface. The local skin turns crimson with hyperemia, and blisters might appear.

To observe the effect of natural moxibustion on asthma patients' immunological function, a study was completed on the observation of 121 patients' soluble leucocyte SIL-2R and T lymphocyte subgroups. Medicinal preparation for natural moxibustion were as follows: using ephedra, asarum, Kansui Radix, corydalis and raw white mustard powder, and cut with ginger juice, a paste was created. Acupoints selected for treatment included *Feishu* (肺俞 BL13), *Fengmen* (风门 BL12) and *Dingchuan* (定喘 EX-B1); and for the relaxing period, *Feishu* (肺俞 BL13), *Gaohuang* (膏肓 BL38) and *Shenshu* (肾俞 BL23). Results indicated that the serum levels of SIL-2R were higher than that of the normal group, while CD+4 levels and CD+4/CD+8 ratios were also higher. After the treatment of natural moxibustion, patients' SIL-2R levels became lowered, as well as the CD+4 levels and CD+4/CD+8 ratios, thus the change of SIL-2R was obviously related to CD+4 T lymphocytes. It was suggested that natural moxibustion affected the asthma mechanism through the adjustment of T lymphocyte activation. (Lai *et al.*, 2000).

Other experiments revealed that natural moxibustion could obviously lower asthma patients' plasma substance P (SP), raise blood activation and content of the intestinal peptide VIP. Such effects are not observed in regular acupuncture therapy. Compared with acupuncture, natural moxibustion had the advantage of being simple to operate and needing only a short treatment time. It was particularly suitable for treating large numbers of asthma patients (Dai *et al.*, 2001). In one clinical study natural moxibustion was found to have an effective rate of up to 87.5%. Patients' plasma cGMP level did not show any clear difference, but plasma cAMP and cAMP/cGMP levels became much higher (Yang *et al.*, 2003).

To observe factors such as age, course of disease and the nature of disease, that might affect the result of treatment of asthma using natural moxibustion, a large study on the therapeutic effects of the treatment of 1330 asthma patients using natural moxibustion had been completed. Acupoints selected were *Feishu* (肺俞 BL13) and *Xinshu* (心俞 BL15). Medicines used for the natural moxibustion included white mustard seeds 12%, fried white mustard seeds 18%, asarum 30%, corydalis 15%, Kansui Radix 15% and Chinese Eaglewood 10%, mixed with ginger juice to make a cake of 2.5 cm by 0.5 cm. Before applying the cakes on the acupoints, acupuncturists used fresh ginger slice to rub on the acupoints to produce hyperemia. The cakes were retained for at least two hours, and up to 24 hours before they were taken off. The therapeutic results were better for young patients under twenty. The duration of the course of asthma did not have obvious impact on the therapeutic effect (Cai *et al.*, 1992).

9.3 Treating Asthma with Suppurative Moxibustion

Suppurative moxibustion refers to the application of moxibustion by placing a moxa cone directly on the selected accupoint, whereby local tissue became scalded and undergoes suppuration, thus producing long term acupuncture stimulation effects. In general, the key to achieving therapeutic effect of suppuration depends on whether or not the "moxibustion sore" will appear after moxibustion (Sun, 2002).

Suppurative moxibustion is a common practice in treating bronchial asthma. Since ancient times, there has been sophisticated timing for suppurative moxibustion treatment between in relation to seasonal changes as the beginning or end of summer. One study divided 96 cases of bronchial asthma patients into four therapeutic groups, namely: suppurative moxibustion group, non-suppurative moxibustion group, local anesthetic moxibustion group, and random (season unrelated) moxibustion group. Acupoints selected were *Daizhui* (大椎 DU GV14) and *Feishu* (肺俞 BL13). For the suppurative moxibustion group, the moxa cone used has a diameter of 0.5 cm and height 0.5 cm. Moxibustion was carried out once on alternate days, after which the moxibustion sore was protected with dressing, which was changed every day. For the non-suppurative moxibustion group, no dressing was applied. For the local anesthetic group, Lidocaine was injected for subcutaneous anesthesia, after which suppurative moxibustion was applied. For the random moxibustion group: treatment was similar to that of suppurative moxibustion in which the therapeutic period was carried out in springtime. Results showed the effective rates/total effective rate of the suppurative moxibustion group was 34.1%/63.7%, for the spring moxibustion group the rates were 23.5%/70.6%. For the local anesthetic moxibustion group, the rates were 47.4%/63.2%. All groups were obviously doing better than the non-suppurative moxibustion groups, while there was no obvious difference between the three suppurative moxibustion groups themselves. This study suggested that (1) the therapeutic effect of suppurative moxibustion on bronchial asthma is apparently higher than that of the non-suppurative moxibustion; and (2) there is no seasonal difference in the application of suppurative moxibustion (Hong *et al.*, 1992).

To study the possible immunological mechanisms of action related to bronchial asthma in response to suppurative moxibustion, researchers conducted blood tests and found that bronchial asthma patients had higher plasma total IgE and higher peripheral blood basophil granulocytes compared with normal people, while their plasma cAMP levels were lower. After applying suppurative moxibustion on *Feishu* (肺俞 BL13) and *Daizhui* (大椎 DU GV14), their plasma IgE levels and the absolute counting of basophil granulocytes became remarkably lowered, and the plasma cAMP levels became higher. Those treated with non-suppurative moxibustion did not show such effects. It should be pointed out that suppurative moxibustion might have achieved a better therapeutic effect through the improvement of immunological functions thus raising the cAMP content. To further explore the effects of suppurative moxibustion on regulating

T lymphocytes, researchers used the classification of OKT$^+$strain cloned antibody to test and measure asthma patients' T lymphocytes. The results revealed that the number of OKT$_3^+$ and OKT$_4^+$ cells in asthma patients did not differ from those of normal people, with OKT$_8^+$ obviously lower and OKT$_4^+$/OKT$_8^+$ ratio higher than those of healthy people. This indicated that asthma patients' elevation of plasma IgE levels may be due to the fact that their OKT$_8^+$ cell subgroup number is too low and their OKT$_4^+$/OKT$_8^+$ ratio is too high. Suppurative moxibustion could increase the number of OKT$_8^+$ cells and lower the OKT$_4^+$/OKT$_8^+$ ratio, while non-suppurative moxibustion did not produce such effects (Hong *et al.*, 1993).

Since suppurative moxibustion in treating asthma could give a better therapeutic effect than simple moxibustion, does that mean that the suppuration caused by such moxibustion is the key factor in improving patients' immune function to give a better result? To find out the relations between the amount of suppuration and the therapeutic effect, researchers divided 86 cases randomly according to the size supportive produced using 9-cone, 6-cone and 3-cones of moxibustion. The result indicated that the 9-cone group produced the largest area of moxibustion sore, and its therapeutic effects was obviously better than the 3-cones group but less so compared with the 6-cone groups.

9.4 Treating Asthma with a Combination of Acupuncture and Cupping Method

The application of acupuncture to *Feishu* (肺俞 BL13), *Fengmen* (风门 BL12) and *Daizhui* (大椎 DU GV14) is a common practice of asthma treatment. After getting the *qi*, needles were retained for 30 min. After the needles were withdrawn, a large size cupping tool was placed between *Daizhui* (大椎 DU GV14) and the two *Feishu* (肺俞 BL13) points, to be retained for 10–15 min. The effective rate of this method was reported to be as high as 85% (Yang Yonqing *et al.*, 1994). To explore its functioning mechanism, after the needling treatment, researchers carried out tests and measurements on patients' saliva, nose secretion, SIgA in phlegm and the content of IgA of peripheral blood lymphocyte PWM taken from the clear fluid on the stimulated culture medium. Results indicated that acupuncture could clearly lower the content of SIgA and the total content of IgA in patients saliva and nose secretion, and effectively control patients' delayed asthma attacks. After treatment with acupuncture, as asthma patients' peripheral blood IL-2R+ became activated, T lymphocytes and acidophil granulocytes obviously decreased. This produced a positive preventive effect on further attacks of allergic asthma. After needling, the patients' peripheral blood CD_4^+ T cells became higher than those before treatment, and much higher than the normal level. Whether or not acupuncture has changed asthma patients' reaction to foreign protein, it remains to be confirmed (Yang *et al.*, 1995).

9.5 Summary and Discussion

The mechanism of treating asthma with acupuncture can be summed up with the following points:

(1) Improving breathing function: acupuncture can increase patients' maximum ventilating capacity, VC, VC1 and FEV1, and lower the resistance of respiratory tract, leading to the relief and control of asthma patient's bronchial spasm.

(2) Adjusting immunological function: acupuncture could lower patients' absolute count of peripheral blood basophil granulocytes, resulting in the degranulation of basophil granulocytes and the level of IgE, or adjust the T lymphocytes activation, thus suppressing the production of IgE and controlling type 1 abnormal reaction by lowering serum SIL-2R and CD_4^+ levels and CD_4^+/CD_8^+ ratios. By lowering serum IL-4 levels, raising INF-r levels, and adjusting the loss of balance in Th1/Th2 subgroup function, acupuncture was able to lower respiratory tract's inflammation and hyperreaction. By lowering patients' SIgA content and total IgA content in their saliva and nose secretion, it could effectively delay patients' onset of asthma reactions.

(3) Adjusting patients' second messenger (cAMP and cGMP) content and proportion: by raising the excitability of patients' sympathetic system, suppressing hyperfunction of the parasympathetic system, and strengthening adrenal cortical function, it raises their plasma cAMP levels and cAMP/cGMP ratios, and lowers plasma cGMP levels, resulting in the relief of bronchial spasms, improvement of ventilation function, and relief from asthma.

As the pathogenesis of asthma is complicated, there is a variety of ways through which we could achieve the satisfactory effect in treating asthma with acupuncture, but all final results were achieved through the relief of bronchial spasms. Apart from this, acupuncture also produce balancing effects on a series of humoral balances which helps to control inflammation.

9.6 Additional Views

Acupuncture experts have clear and conceptually understood about the use of the technique under different circumstances. The basic application is of course related to acute attacks while patients have already developed severe or moderate degrees of asthmatic attack. Acupuncturists are aware of the fact that when an acute attack has already developed, it might not be the best time to start acupuncture. Instead, the technique would best be administered on the earliest indication of the attack, so as to prevent a full-scale attack. Acupuncture, in addition, has long been used as a means to prevent asthmatic attacks months before the likely occurrence. This practice is consistent with the traditional concept of "pre-season prevention" on "treating winter disease with summer intervention" (冬病夏治) and special technical details are recommended.

The "pre-season prevention" in reality involves acupuncture together with moxibustion and the intentional production of burnt ulcers. The slow healing of these artificially produced, suppurative ulcers maintains a continuous stimulation over the selected acupuncture points, which should have the preventive effects maintained. This practice was popular some hundreds of years ago when anti-asthmatic medication was hardly developed. With the introduction of more and better choices of asthmatic drugs, acute control of asthma becomes more effective. Thence the use of the cumbersome moxibustion turned less popular. However, with the recent increase in the incidence of asthma, rising with deteriorating air quality, more application of the pre-season prevention is reappearing. In some major cities, there are community campaigns calling for mass reception of acupuncture and moxibustion in summer, aiming at the prevention of attacks in winter. Acupuncture-moxibustion involves a long process of 2–3 months where the septic ulcers resulting from the moxibustion need daily/frequent cleaning, dressing and other more energetic measures to control the septic spread.

The duration of suppurative acupuncture usually takes 1–2 months after the initiating puncture. The choice of acupuncture points needs to be simple, including: *Daizhui* (大椎 DU GV14), *Feishu* (肺俞 BL13) and *Fengmen* (风门 BL12), which are popularly selected after moxibustion, suppurative ulcer are produced at the puncture sites. The patient and relatives need to be very cooperative and be responsible for the execution of recommended treatment procedures. If the ulcers heal too quickly, additional punctures involving other acupoints should be considered. Overall, about one-third of recipients achieve good improvement. For those patients who experience an annual attack of asthma, an annual treatment is recommended. Such preventive procedures have been traditionally practiced in summer time. However, experts consider that the seasonal preference is unimportant as long as the procedures are designed to prevent the attacks after 2–3 months. There should be little worry about the aftermath of the septic ulcers. The ulcers are shallow, and the sizes are usually limited to below 2.5 cm in diameter. With careful daily dressing healing should be guaranteed. The resulting scars could be obvious but asymptomatic. In case healing is difficult, acupuncturists would recommend the use of antibiotics. If the moxibustion fails to give the satisfactory results, other measures like acupoint injection, other body punctures or acupoint suction, etc., could be added.

Acupuncturists used to warn patients that asthma is a chronic disease, the treatment of which could be difficult and results unpredictable.

Indeed asthmatic patients are facing multiple challenges. In the first place, they usually carry a familial tendency of allergy. Secondly, the over-reaction to immuno-modulating stimulations, going through complicated cellular and molecular activation, is not perfectly understood yet. Thirdly, the environmental factors, like air pollution and food influences, are dramatic initiating factors to the asthmatic attacks. With the consideration of the multiple etiological factors, the healers, either from the traditional or the conventional stream, should acknowledge to their patients that treatment results could be deficient of full responses; they could be partial or even unsatisfactory. Healers should realize that we are facing a pathological condition that is complex and would be an exception if one simple and straightforward treatment modality could uproot the problem. On the contrary, difficulties should be expected, chronicity can be expected and recurrences, even after apparent satisfactory control, are not surprising.

For the benefits of the patients, healers should be prepared to use multiple options of treatment, either supplementing each other or even used simultaneously.

References

Cai, L.N., Chen, Y.L. and Shi, N.Y. (1992) Clinical analysis of 1330 asthma patients by treatment of Medicinal Vesiculation. *Fujian J. Tradit. Chin. Med.* **23**(2), 23–25.

Dai, W. and Lai, X. (2001) The effect of medicinal vesiculation therapy on plasma SP and VIP contents in bronchial asthma patients. *Acupunct. Res.* **26**(2), 134–136.

Feng, J.G., Chen, D.Z. and Cheng, B.H. (1983) Clinical studies of acupuncture treatment of bronchial asthma — the relationship between the plasma cyclic nucleotides and cortisol changes of asthma patients and asthma symptoms relief. *Shanghai J. Tradit. Chin. Med.* **7**, 26–28.

Feng, J.G., Shen, R.B., Chen, D.Z., *et al.* (1983) The effect of acupuncture on respiratory function in bronchial asthma. *Shanghai J. Acupunct. Moxibustion* **1**, 19, 41.

Hong, H.G., Chen, H.P., Yan, H., *et al.* (1993) The influence of purulent moxibustion on immune function in patients with bronchial asthma. *Shanghai J. Acupunct. Moxibustion* **12**(2), 59–60.

Hong, H.G., Yan, H., Chen, H.P., *et al.* (1992) Treatment of bronchial asthma by suppurative moxibustion — analysis of influencing factors. *Shanghai J. Acupunct. Moxibustion* **2**, 5.

Lai, X.S., Li, Y.M., Zhang, J.W., *et al.* (2000) Effects of medicinal vesiculation on serum soluble IL-2 receptor and T lymphocyte subsets in patients of asthma. *Chin. Acupunct. Moxibustion* **1**, 33–35.

Sun, G.J. (2002) *Science of Acupuncture and Moxibustion.* People's Medical Publishing House, pp. 533.

Yang, Y.Q., Chen, H.P., Wang, R.Z., *et al.* (1995) The influence of acupuncture treatment on the active cell number of T lymphocytes and eosinophils on the peripheral blood of patients with asthma. *Shanghai J. Acupunct. Moxibustion* **20**(2), 68–70.

Yang, Y.Q., Chen, H.P., Zhao, C.Y., *et al.* (1995) The study of acupuncture for allergic asthma patients of immunomodulation of mucosal SIgA. *Acupunct. Res.* **20**(2), 68–70.

Yang, J.J. and Lai, X.S. (2003) Research on therapeutic effects and mechanism of treatment of bronchial asthma by medicinal vesiculation. *J. Tradit. Chin. Med.* **23**(4), 7–8.

Zhang, Z., Ji, X., Xue, L., *et al.* (2005) Clinical observation on acupuncture for treatment of bronchial asthma at acute stage. *Chin. Acupunct. Moxibustion* **25**(3), 158–160.

Chapter 10

Acupuncture for Joint Pain
— Acupuncture Treatment on Rheumatoid Arthritis

Abstract

Rheumatoid Arthritis (RA) is primarily an autoimmune disease, affecting multiple joints. The symptomatic manifestations include joint stiffness in the morning, painful swollen joints and functional disorders. The mild cases suffer from chronic joint pain and functional deteriorations, while severe and burnt-out cases become invalid. To date, therapeutic medicine provides the main core of treatment for RA. Usually, only non-specific treatment, such as non-steroidal anti-inflammatory drugs or adrenal glucocorticoids could be effective. The non-responsive cases might need specific drugs, such as penicillamine, or other immunosuppressants like Levamisole. According to Chinese Medicine Concept RA reflects the occurrence of "wind", "cold", "dampness" and "heat" lying stagnant within the meridians and circulatory channels, thus causing disharmony between "qi" and "blood", which gives rise to pain, swelling and dysfunction. Acupuncture lifts the disharmony and has been used as a treatment method for RA over a long time. Recent clinical reports are also plentiful.

Keywords: Rheumatoid Arthritis; Moxibustion.

10.1 Simple Acupuncture as a Treatment Method

The acupoints selected are primarily around the four limbs, especially around the joints. One study selected primarily ST 36, CV 4, GV 3 and BL 23 supported by ancillary points: TE 15LI 4, TE 4, LI 5 and SI 5 in the upper limbm and SP 6, ST 41, LR 3, KI 6, and BL 62 in the lower limb. Acupuncture was given once daily and 20 days composed one treatment course. Patients received at least one and a half treatment courses, and not more than eight. One hundred and five cases of RA patients were included in a study; the results were as follows: (1) before treatment the RA patients' serum IgG, IgM, and erythrocyte sedimentation rates were all higher than normal. After acupuncture treatment, data were all lowered; (2) using Chinese Medicine concepts to analyze the results, it was found that the improvements had no bearing on specific physiological presentations; and (3) studying the relationship between the treatment course and effects, it was found that there was no significant difference between three courses treatment and four–six courses treatment. However seven–eight courses treatment seemed to give better effect (Wu *et al.*, 1990).

"Acupuncture taking advantage of the hottest summer days" (顺势伏针法) is based on the compilation of the experiences of famous acumoxi practitioner, Professor Xi Yongjiang (奚永江教授). Acupuncture treatment for RA could combine the holistic with the local concept. Holistic treatment relies primarily on the GV and BL 28, which aim at warming and supplementing, while the local treatment acupoints aim to control pain. Clinical studies found that acupuncture could relieve soft tissue and synovial membrane hyperemia and edema. This was proven in RA animal models where inflammation control was obvious in cellular and molecular studies (Gao *et al.*, 2000). Acupuncture was also shown to be working through immunological modulations (Huang *et al.*, 1995).

10.2 Moxibustion Treatment Method

Moxibustion is a popular method of treatment for RA. Special herbs have been used during moxibustion; examples include ginger, garlic, musk, corydalis, white mustard, cinnamon and asarum. One study recruited 65 outpatients with RA. They were randomly divided into moxibustion group and medication group. In the moxibustion group, the acupoints selected included GV 14, BL 11, BL 17, BL 20 and BL 23. Moxibustion was given with three large moxa cones, until local skin turned red and moist. Moxibustion was applied once every two days, 30 days comprising a treatment course, and observation was made after six courses. The control group used oral administration of Meloxicam tablets, 75 mg, once daily. The evaluation for treatment effect included the follows: (1) joint pain, pressure pain; (2) morning stiffness; (3) joint swelling; (4) general fatigue; and (5) erythrocyte sedimentation rate (ESR); etc. The results showed that in the moxibustion group, out of the 33 cases, 19 enjoyed good effects, 10 enjoyed effects, and the total effective rate was 87.9%. For the medication group, out of 32 cases, 12 had good effects, 9 enjoyed effects, and the total effective rate was 65.5%. Apparently the moxibustion group was better than medication group.

The application of ginger moxibustion for the treatment of RA in 94 cases of RA patients randomly divided into ginger group (31 cases), smokeless ginger group (33 cases), and control group using penicillamine (30 cases). The point selection of the treatment groups was as follows: (1) CV 17, CV 12, CV 6, CV 8, ST 36; and (2) BL 17, BL 18, BL 20, GV 4. Two groups of points were used alternately. The moxa cone was placed on top of a ginger slice, which protected the skin from burns. For both treatment groups, treatment was carried out once daily, 50 times comprising a treatment course. For the control group using oral administration of penicillamine, treatment time was the same as the treatment groups. Observations were made before and after treatment for the clinical improvements, erythrocyte sedimentation, rheumatoid factors, immune globulin, and complement, etc. The results were as follows: the smokeless group had a total effective rate of 81.8%, ginger 80.6%, penicillamine control group 72.0%, and there was no significant difference between the three groups (Yang *et al.*, 2007).

Sixty-three RA patients were divided into three groups (aconite cake moxibustion group 15 cases, aconite cake mild smoke moxibustion group 16 cases, and ginger moxibustion group 32 cases) for the analysis of clinical results. The results were as follows: the total effective rate of aconite cake moxibustion group was 93.33%, aconite cake with mild smoke moxibustion group, 81.25%, and ginger moxibustion group, 93.75%. There was no significant difference among the three groups (Wang *et al.*, 2001).

10.3 Temperature Acupuncture

Temperature acupuncture is to enhance the acupuncture effects. Acu-points primarily selected were CV 4, CV 6, ST 36, BL 18, BL 20 and BL 23, to be matched with local points of the joint affection area. Twenty-nine RA patients were treated this way, and were matched with a control group of 28 cases. From the results, it was found that the clinical treatment effect of acupuncture and simple moxibustion was significantly better than that of the control group, with a total effective rate of 86.21% and 57.14% respectively. Acupuncture and simple moxibustion significantly reduced RA patients' joint pain, swelling, handicap index, morning stiffness, and 20-meter walking time, and increased gripping power; results were significantly better than the control group. At the same time, the patients' serum ESR, RF, CRP, IgA, IgG and IgM levels were all lowered. The milder the condition and the shorter the course of disease, the better the responses observed (Liu *et al.*, 2006).

A comparison study between acupuncture with moxibustion and pure acupuncture for treatment of RA, using CV 4, CV 6, ST 36, BL 18, BL 23 and BL 20, matched with acupoints selected from around the affected joints. The control group applied pure acupuncture treatment. The results showed adding moxibustion total boosted up the effective rate (85.86), which was significantly higher than that of the pure acupuncture group (56.47) (Jin, 2007).

Adding moxibustion on ST 36, CV 4, BL 18, BL 23, ST 33, SP 10, CV 14, BL 11 and LI 11 achieved better results with the hemorrheological indices, Superoxide Dismutase (SOD) activity, and lipid peroxidase (Lpo) level (Li, 1999).

10.4 Electro-Acupuncture (EA) Method

(1) EA was used for treatment on 147 patients divided were randomly into three groups (each with 49 cases). Group A used the acupoints of both hands, including GV 14, TE 5, GB 34, BL 60, ST 31 and GB 33; and other acu-points over both hand fingers, including LI 11, GV 3, LI 10, ST 35 and GB 39. The two groups of points were used alternately. EA with continuous waves, at frequency of 60 Hz, was given for 30 min, twice daily. Ten days form a treatment course, and two courses was the standard. Medication used was cefotamine, once daily, ten days as a treatment course, totaling two courses. Group B just applied pure EA treatment, using the similar acupoints. Group C just used the medication cefotamine. The results of the trial showed that the total effective rate of Group A (97.96%) was significantly better than B and C (46.94%, 42.86%). All three methods significantly reduced the level of Rheumatoid Factor (Rf), Antistrptolysin O (ASO), C-Reactive Protein (CRP) in patients' serum, of which the effect of Group A was still better (Liu *et al.*, 2003).

(2) Other studies indicated that EA applied on ST 36 could increase the content of CS and glucocorticoid resistance (GCR) of the RA rat

model (Yu *et al.*, 2002). EA also significantly reduced the phagocytic IL-1 and spleen cell IL-6 activity (Wang *et al.*, 2001).

10.5 "Fire Needling"

The application of heated needles on *ashi* points, i.e. directly approaching the focci, as a treatment for RA, is also popular. A study on the puncture effects of *ashi* points between the neck and spine on 41 RA patients was done. The *ashi* points were matched with TE 14, LI 15, LI 14; and LI 12, LI 11 and LI 10. For those suffering from wrist pain, the matching acupoints included TE 4, LI 5 and SI 5. Those suffering from lower limbs joint pain, the *ashi* points were matched with EX-LE 5, ST 34, ST 36 and GB 34. Those suffering from ankle joint pain were matched with ST 41 and GB 40. The control group used the same *ashi* puncture treatment together with oral administration of medication consisting of penicillamine, CTX and ibuprofen. The results showed a total effective rate of 91.11% in the treatment group while only 71.79% was recorded in the group. One-year follow-up also indicated that the risk of recurrence in the treatment group was also less than the control (Wu *et al.*, 2002).

10.6 Discussion

In Chinese Medicine concept, RA could be understood as belonging to "limb analgesia" category. The cause of "limb analgesia" could be "wind", "coldness", "humidity" or "heat"; such causes could well be not apparent or hidden. Using acupuncture for treatment carries the principle of re-establishing the blocked meridian channels. With this complex demand a multitude of puncture methodology should be considered. When coldness and humidity were observed, warm needling, moxibustion, electrical puncturing or cupping with bloodletting could be considered. For heat and humidity, more simple choices of acupoints with bloodletting, particularly those known to release "wind", like *Feng-chi* (風池 GB20), *Feng-fu* (風府 DU16) or *Tai-chong* (太沖 LR3) could be selected. When joint swelling or joint effusion is observed, acupoint injection into the tender spots could be advisable. Agents used for acupoint injection are those known to have stimulating effects on circulation promotion. Examples are *Angelica sinensis* and *Danshen* extracts. The depth of needling should be evaluated according to the presence of coldness or heat. For the former, needling depth should be deeper than latter.

A good simple practice for the mild type of rheumatoid attack is the simple application of cupping. After the first cupping application, when a deep hemorrhagic mark results, subsequent cupping could add extracts of herbal agents known to release "wind". Such agents include *Hai-feng-teng* (海風藤 *caulis piperis kadsurae*), *Gui-zhi* (桂枝 *Ramulus Cinnamomi*) and *Hong-hua* (紅花 *Carthamus tinctorius L.*).

Finally, a look at a carefully planned clinical study will be beneficial.

A group of rheumatologists have conducted a clinical trial on rheumatoid patients already maintained on various doses of steroidal preparations.

In planning a randomized controlled trial of acupuncture, a pilot study was conducted in 2006, using validated outcome measures to assess the feasibility of the protocol, and to obtain preliminary data on the efficacy and tolerability of three different forms of acupuncture treatment as an adjunct for the treatment of chronic pain in patients with RA.

The study employed randomized, prospective, double-blind, placebo-controlled trial to evaluate the effect of EA, traditional Chinese acupuncture (TCA) and sham acupuncture (Sham) in patients with RA. All patients received 20 sessions over a period of ten weeks. Six acupuncture points were chosen. Primary outcome was the changes in the pain score. Secondary outcomes included the changes in the American College of Rheumatology (ACR) core disease measures, disease activity score using the 28 joint counts (DAS 28) score, and the number of patients who achieved ACR 20 at week ten.

From 80 eligible patients, 36 patients with mean age of 58 ± 10 years and disease duration of 9.3 ± 6.4 years were recruited. Twelve patients were randomized to each group. Twelve, ten and seven patients from the EA, TCA and Sham group respectively completed the study at 20 weeks ($p < 0.03$); all except one of the premature dropouts were due to lack of efficacy. At week ten, the pain score remained unchanged in all three groups. The number of tender joints was significantly reduced for the EA and TCA groups. Physician's global score was significantly reduced for the EA group and patient's global score was significantly reduced for the TCA group. All the outcomes except patient's global score remained unchanged in the Sham group.

The conclusion of the pilot study has allowed a number of recommendations to be made to facilitate the design of a large-scale trial, which in turn will help to clarify the existing evidence based on acupuncture for RA (Tam and Leung, 2007).

References

Gao, H., Liu, G.P. and Huang, D.J. (2000) Morphological observations of acupuncture treatment of rheumatoid arthritis in rats. *Shanghai J. Acupunct. Moxibustion* **19**(6), 37–38.

Huang, D.J., Luo, Y.Z., Zhou, Z.K., *et al.* (1995) Effects of moxibustion and needling on erythrocytic immune function and contents of plasma cortisol in rats of experimental rheumatoid arthritis. *Chin. Acupunct. Moxibustion* **15**(6), 25–28.

Jin, Y.J. (2007) Clinical observation of warm acupuncture treatment for 56 patients with rheumatoid arthritis. **3**, 140.

Li, L. (1999) Clinical observation of warm acupuncture treatment for 35 patients with rheumatoid arthritis. *J. Tianjin Coll. Tradit. Chin. Med.* **18**(3), 31–32.

Liu, J.Z. and Ju, Y.L. (2007) Clinical observation of warm acupuncture treatment of rheumatoid arthritis. *Shanghai J. Acupunct. Moxibustion* **3**, 140.

Liu, L.G., Liu, L., Luo, S.D., *et al.* (2003) Therapeutic effect of electroacupuncture combined with medicine on acute rheumatoid arthritis. *Chin. Acupunct. Moxibustion* **23**(12), 712–714.

Tam, L.-S., Leung, P.-C., Li, T.K., Zhang, L. and Li, E.K. (2007) Acupuncture in the treatment of rheumatoid arthritis: A double-blind controlled pilot study. *BMC Complem. Altern. Med.* **7**, 35.

Wang, R.H. and Yang, J.B. (2001) The influence of electro-acupuncture on the activity of IL-1 and IL-6 of adjuvant-induced arthritis in rats. *J. Shaanxi Coll. Tradit. Chin. Med.* **24**(4), 43–45.

Wang, W.M., Chen, H.P., Yang, Z., *et al.* (2001) The treatment of rheumatoid arthritis by different indirect moxibustions. *Shanghai J. Acupunct. Moxibustion* **20**(2), 9–11.

Wu, H.D., Tian, W.H. and Fu, G.B. (2002) Fire-needle treatment of 45 patients with rheumatoid arthritis. *Shanxi J. Tradit. Chin. Med.* **18**(5), 40–41.

Wu, F., Ji, Q.S., Wang, J., *et al.* (1990) Clinical observation of acupuncture treatment for 105 patients with rheumatoid arthritis. *Liaoning J. Tradit. Chin. Med.* **9**, 40–42.

Yang, Z., Song, Y.W., Cheng, L.P., *et al.* (2007) Clinical observation of rheumatoid arthritis treatment by the smoke-free moxibustion divided by ginger. *J. Hebei Tradit. Chin. Med. Pharmacol.* **22**(1), 28–30.

Yu, S.G., Tang, Y. and Liu, Y.X. (2002) Effect of electroacupuncture of "Zusanli" on plasma corticosterone content and glucocorticosteroid receptor affinity and concentration of rheumatoid arthritis rats. *Acupunct. Res.* **27** (3), 205–209.

Chapter 11

Acupuncture for Bladder Control — Treatment for Urethral Syndrome in the Women

Abstract

Urethral Syndrome (US) mainly refers to the sensitivity of the lower urinal tract, presenting as urinary frequency, urgency, dysuria and lower abdomen distension. Neither organic pathology on the bladder or urethra nor bacterial infection could be detected. Female Urethral Syndrome (FUS) mainly affects middle age and paramenopausal women; hence it is also labeled as FUS.

Current research maintains that the disease is related to subclinical: infection, urethral obstruction, psychological influences, neurofunctional disorder, immunological imbalance, urination habit, aging, and sexual life. Clinical factors might include physical fatigue, respiratory tract infection, change of weather, drinking and sexual habits. Apart from urinary frequency, urgency, dysuria, suprapubic pain, incontinence, tenesmus, post-micturition pain, adverse sexual activities, are also observed.

To date, there is yet no consensus understanding of FUS with regard to its etiological, pathology, and treatment. However, FUS is not a fatal condition although the affected might suffer from a severely disturbed quality of life. After years of clinical disappointment in spite of standard management, acupuncture has been endorsed as an option of treatment.

Keywords: Female Urethral Syndrome; Bladder Function; Urinary Tract.

11.1 Needling and Moxibustion Used Together

Urethral Syndrome (US) mainly refers to the sensitivity of the lower urinal tract, presenting as urinary frequency, urgency, dysuria and lower abdomen distension. No bladder or urethral organic pathology could be detected nor is there bacterial infection. FUS mainly affects middle age and para-menopausal women, hence it is also labeled as Female Urethral Syndrome (FUS) (Schmidt, 1985). According to the clinical characteristics of FUS, Chinese Medicine practitioners maintained that FUS is a manifestation of kidney insufficiency. The diagnosis of FUS starts with the exclusion of organic pathology and infection of the urinary tract. To date, hospital treatment includes the following: (1) surgical operation, which can be used to expand the urethra or to induce the urethral sphincter, and other operations include urethrotomy and cryotheraphy; (2) medication, which includes antibiotics, female hormonal treatment, Triamcinolone, tranquilizers, calcium ion isolators (and prostate glandinhibitor for the male); and (3) psychological treatment and biofeedback rehabilitation (Zhang and Jin, 1995; Li, 1998). Acupuncture treatment is primarily intended to supplement the kidney insufficiency through the warming of the *yang* meridians by stimulating CV 6, CV 4, KI 12, KI 11, ST 28, SP 6, and KI 3; GV 4, BL 22, BL 23, BL 24, BL 29, BL 35 and BL 39. Two groups of points were used alternately. Three to four points were selected every time, during the treatment. Long needles and deep insertions were applied to BL 29 and BL 35, producing acuesthesia projected towards the direction of lower abdomen. Needle was retained at CV 1 for 20 min. In the control group, oral administration of a proprietor drugs viz. Hu Qian Lie Pian was used. One treatment course consisted of ten acupuncture sessions and 1–2 courses were the standard. The treatment effect (88.3%) of the acupuncture group was better than control group (28%). The long term treatment effect (half a year to one year) of acupuncture could reach 79.1%. Acupuncture also increased urinary flow on an average increase of 4.9 ml/s, while the control group suffered an average decline of 1.3 ml/s. The urethral sphincter pressure is another means to illustrate the effect of acupuncture. The acupuncture group enjoyed a relaxation of 18 cmH$_2$O, while the control group increased an average of 9.8 cmH$_2$O (Zheng *et al.*, 1996).

11.2 Comparison between Electro-Acupuncture (EA) and Hand Needling

Eighty-nine female patients were randomly divided into EA group (54 cases), and hand needling group (35 cases), and the acupoint selection was as follows: (1) CV 3, KI 12, ST 28, SP 6; and (2) BL 23, BL 29, BL 35, BL 40. The two groups of points could be used alternately. Treatment was applied once every other day, and ten treatments were taken as a course. After one treatment course, an evaluation was made according to the International Urine Control Association Urinary Handicap Symptoms, and the Living Qualities evaluation was made before and after treatment. The results showed that both groups enjoyed more normal urination after treatment, but the functional scores between the two groups did not show significant difference. The EA group gave early improvement of 51.8%, higher than that of manual needling, which gave only 17.1% of early improvement (Chen *et al.*, 2005). At the same time EA improved the bladder volume, but did not affect the patients' urinary flow rate (Chen *et al.*, 2006).

11.3 Comparison of the Treatment Effects of Different EA Parameters

One hundred and eight cases of FUS patients were randomly divided into a continuous wave group, rarefaction wave group, and an intermittent wave group to carry out EA treatment, each with 36 cases. The points selected were as follows: BL 35 and BL 29. The results were as follows:

(1) For the rarefaction wave group the effective rate reached 63.89%, and the total effective rate reached 80.56%. The improvements were significantly higher than the continuous waves group (44.44%, 72.22%) and intermittent waves group (50%, 72.22%).
(2) With regard to lowering of the urethral sphincter pressure, abdomen pressure, and functional urethral length, the rarefaction wave group gave the most outstanding results. Urinary flow, however, was not affected by any of the waveforms.
(3) The intermittent waves group had the least effects on the relaxation of bladder pressure, while the continuous waves and rarefaction wave groups better results than the intermittent waves (Shen and Shen, 2003).

11.4 Treatment Effect of Single Acupoints and Special Points

Simple puncturing on BL 35 three times may improve the urethral problems of a patient with FUS, as assessed with the International Prostate Symptom Score (I-PSS). Applying acupuncture on GB 30 three times could only partially improve FUS symptoms. The improvement on other urinary disorders is not as good as BL 35. Moreover, accumulative effects with repeated punctures on specific acupuncture points have been demonstrated.

When EA was applied on KI 12 and ST 28, requiring acuesthesia to transmit to urethral orifice, it could increase the pressure of the bladder detrusor, thus improving urine flow rate (Shen and Shen, 2004).

Using "Four sacral needles" treatment method to treat female pressure urinary incontinence, the treatment effect is superior to general acupuncture method treatment (point selection by pattern differentiation). The "Four sacral needles" needling method refers to two upper needles near the edge of the sacral bone, corresponding to the level of posterior sacral foramina. The lower needles are located 0.5 cun lateral to the end of the coccyx. EA uses continuous waves at 1.67–1.83 Hz frequency, lasting for 60 min. During the EA, the pelvic diaphragm reacts with rhythmic upward contractions. Treatment was given once daily, and the number of treatments depends on the responses. Electro stimulation was directly applied to excite the pudendal nerve, inducing pelvic bottom muscles to have rhythmic contractions, thereby strengthening pelvic bottom muscle to improve urine control faculty; moreover, it follows that the pelvic diaphragm contraction together with the urethral sphincter stimulation could improve the urinary control mechanisms, and this option could be better than some other general acupuncture method (Wang *et al.*, 2006).

11.5 Mechanism of Action of Acupuncture and Moxibustion on the Modulation of Bladder Function

The nervous control of the urinary bladder has three kinds of components: sympathetic input, parasympathetic involvement, and vicerosensory influence. Of these, the sympathetic nerves come from T11 to L2 of the spinal cord; parasympathetic nerve comes from S2 to S4; and the vicerosensory involvement includes a complex system of somatic pain perception via the spinal cord and splanchnic-connection (Zhou, 1996).

Normal urination is a kind of nervous reflex activity controlled consciously through central reflex mechanism of the brain and spinal cord. Adults could voluntarily regulate and control urination. When the bladder is filled up to a certain extent, the bladder wall mechanicoreceptors, which are stretched to a certain threshold tension, transmit an excitement message upwards to the sacral cord centre in the spine and the connation centre in the cerebral cortex where urination desire is initiated. When circumstances permit, the urination centre on the spine will issue urination instruction downward, reaching the sacral cord via the pelvic nerve, and the detrusor contracts, at the same time hypogastric nerve and pudendal nerves are inhibited, making initiating the relaxation of bladder sphincter and pelvic diaphragm muscle, thus opening the gate and produce urination. The sympathetic nerve has a negative feedback effect on urination. When the intravesical pressure rises, sympathetic nerve becomes excited, inhibiting detrusor to contract or relax, thus increasing the storage capacity of the bladder. At the time of urination, the excitement impulse of the sympathetic nerve will stop (Zhou, 1996).

The functional abnormality of the bladder is mainly manifested in the abnormal function of urine storage and urination, and the appearance of such symptoms as dysuria, retention of urine, incontinence, urinary frequency, urgency, and urethralgia. Pathologies of the kidney, ureter, urethra, prostate and bladder itself could all influence the function of bladder, causing numerous symptoms. The influence of acupuncture on the bladder function has already been revealed through a large number of clinical observations and animal experiments, and the modulating effect takes a duplex direction.

11.6 Clinical Studies

To study the treatment effect of acumoxi on urethral high pressure of female with US, an experiment was conducted in which 93 cases of women suffering from high urethral pressure were randomly divided into acupuncture treatment group (56 cases) and medication control group (37 cases). In the treatment group, two groups of acupoints with alternate application where utilized. The first group took CV 6, CV 4, KI 12, KI 11, ST 28, SP 6 and KI 3. The second group took GV 4, BL 22, BL 23, BL 24, BL 29, BL 35 and BL 39. Each time 3–4 points were used, all applied with lifting-thrusting twirling-turning reinforcement. For BL 35 and BL 29, long needles were used for deep insertion and were retained for 20 min. Re-examination was carried out after 1–2 treatment courses. The control group was treated with proprietary Chinese Medicine. It was found that after acupuncture, the treatment group achieved a total effective rate of 88%, the maximal urethral sphincter pressure dropped 24.3 cmH$_2$O. The highest urine flow rate on the average increased 4.5 ml/s. For the control group, the total effective rate was only 30%, the highest urethral sphincter pressure on the average increased 6.8 cmH$_2$O, and there was no significant change in the maximal urine flow rate. Further analysis found that patients' clinical symptomatic improvements were significantly related to the decline of the urethral sphincter pressure (Wang *et al.*, 1997; Deng, 1987; Tao and Ren, 1994).

11.7 The Central Neurological Influence of Acupuncture on Modulation of Bladder Function

(1) When acupuncture was applied to a rabbit's BL 28 and BL 23, the posterior hypothalamic region and the reticular formation of the medulla oblongata unit were found to respond actively. Acupuncture on control points did not have similar influence. The rhythmic contraction of the bladder and the bladder contraction induced by acupuncture followed the neurological activities, and the application of atropine inhibited the contractions. Injection of sodium thiopentone also produced direct inhibitory effects on the reticular formation, thereby stopping the needling effects. Apparently, the afferent acupuncture message is related to the reticular formation, and needling could modulate bladder function via the urination centre (Wu *et al.*, 1982).

(2) When acupuncture was applied to the rabbit's BL 32, leading to the increase of intravesical pressure, the midbrain was involved in this process. It was presumed that the midbrain could be integrating the messages at a high central position, when acupuncture was performed integrated (Zhang and Zhang, 1985).

Application of acupuncture to a cat's BL 32 also increased the intravesical pressure, and lowered the urination threshold value. In the septal area and preoptic area of the brain, unit discharges related to the bladder function during the needling could be recorded (Zhang *et al.*, 1985a). Electro-stimulation of rabbit's dorsal pontine bladder contraction centre raised bladder pressure to 24 mmH_2O; needling BL 32 increased bladder pressure to 30 mmH_2O. When both stimulations were applied simultaneously bladder pressure increased to 60 mmH_2O. When the area was damaged by bilateral electrolysis, it was found that the needling effect reached only 47% of the value before damage. If damage was done on the anterior part of pontine urination centre a significant decline of the needling effect was observed. When needling was applied to control acupoints no such changes were observed (Zhang *et al.*, 1987; 1985b).

In short, both clinical and animal studies indicated that acupuncture treatment had a duplex modulation effect on bladder function:

(1) Central modulation mechanism: the mechanism involved cortex, mid-brain, pons and sacral cord urination center.

(2) Lowering urethral pressure: acupuncture lowered urethral sphincter pressure, increased the maximal urine flow and occlusive pressure, lowered urination threshold, abdominal pressure, and relaxed the pelvic diaphragm, urethral sphincter muscle, and bladder detrusor to accommodate better urine storage.

(3) The clinical results therefore were lowered urination frequency, facilitated urination, better control of urination, and prevention of incontinence.

The modulation effects of acupuncture on bladder function show acupoint specificity. SP 6 has a better duplex modulation effect on detrusor pressure; CV 3 and ST 36 are conducive to increase abdominal pressure; the main manifestation of BL 23 on bladder function is on its inhibitory effects; and BL 32 is good for increasing intravesical pressure.

11.8 Additional Views

Women are prone to the pathophysiology of uncontrolled urination which could be interpreted as incontinence or failure to hold urine. Women who are prone to this ailment are either elderly or belong to the multipara group who has given birth to more than two children. This group of women have weakened pelvic diaphragm, possibly combined with changes in the angulation between the urethra and urinary bladder. Treatment of this abnormal pathophysiology could rely on short term or long term strengthening of the pelvic diaphragm. One most effective option would be the direct stimulation of the bladder sphincter centre at the spinal cord level. This is what the neurosurgeons in collaborations with the urologist are attempting to do by implanting an electrical device in the spinal canal at the high lumbar level. This device gives either regular or periodic stimulation to the spinal cord to induce sphincteric tightening.

Acupuncturists commonly choose four acupuncture points at abdominal levels and sacral levels in the treatment of incontinence. The resulting mechanism could possibly be the activation of the sphincteric centers via some afferent sensory pathways. Modern acupuncturists of today advocate the use of electrical acupuncture for this problem. If observations on the results indicate better results, it might be an indirect indication that the mechanism of action probably works through the sphincteric nuclei in the spinal cord.

As a rule, treatment for this condition, either using bioengineering technology (spinal stimulator) or with acupuncture, is not always effective. Even if improvement is observed, the results could be partial and transient. For those who do not really suffer because of the urination sensitivity, probably they could patiently wait for a natural improvement, which does occur. For those who suffer much, they may choose to receive implant treatment. Before making the decision of receiving the invasive treatment, the patients could first try acupuncture, which probably works through similar mechanisms. If electrical acupuncture gives good results, electrical device implantation might be as effective.

References

Chen, Y.L., Ha, L.P. and Cen, J. (2005) Comparative observation on therapeutic effects of electroacupuncture and manual acupuncture on female urethral syndrome. *Chin. Acupunct. Moxibustion* 25(6), 425–426.

Chen, Y.L., Cen, J. and Hou, W.G. (2006) Comparative study on the effects of electroacupuncture plus hand-acupuncture and simple hand-acupuncture on bladder volume in female urethral syndrome patients. *Acupunct. Res.* 31(2), 116–118.

Deng, C.L. (1994) Exploration of specific points for adjusting bladder function. *Shanghai J. Acupunct. Moxibustion* z1, 66–67.

Li, Y.Y. (1998) Urethral syndrome: It's hard to say for women. *Med. Health Care* 1, 16.

Schmidt, R.A. (1985) The urethral syndrome. *Urol. Clin. North Am.* 12(2), 349–354.

Shen, D.Y. and Shen, P.F. (2003) Clinical research on treating hypertonic pressure of FUS with different electroacupuncture waveform. *Liaoning J. Tradit. Chin. Med.* 30(11), 923–924.

Shen, D.Y. and Shen, P.F. (2004) Clinical study on effects of acupuncture of Dahe and Shuidao points on female urethral syndrome of inertia vesica-urinaria type. *Acupunct. Res.* 29(2), 153–155.

Tao, Z.L. and Ren, W.Q. (1994) Research of neuroanatomy mechanism of acupuncture on "Guan Yuan Yu," "Pangguang Yu" for the treatment of disorders of the urinary system. *Acupunct. Res.* z1, 66–67.

Wang, S.Y., Zhen, H.T. and Huang, C. (1997) Research of acupuncture to reduce the female urethral syndrome in patients with high urethral pressure. *Shanghai J. Acupunct. Moxibustion* 16(2), 4–5

Wang, S.Y., Chen, G.M. and Li, L.H. (2006) "Four sacral needles" therapy for female stress incontinence. *Shanghai J. Acupunct. Moxibustion* 25(5), 13–15.

Wu, D.Z., Yang, L.P. and Deng, C.L. (1982) The impact of acupuncture on the back of the hypothalamus and medulla oblongata micturition center and bladder function. *Chin. Acupunct. Moxibustion* 5, 15.

Zhang, Z.X. and Zhang, H. (1985) Influence of acupuncture on micturition center of the midbrain and bladder function. *Chin. Acupunct. Moxibustion* 6, 31.

Zhang, H., Zhang, Z.X. and Wu, D.Z. (1985a) Influence of acupuncture on the unit discharge of preoptic area and septal area and bladder function. *Shanghai J. Acupunct. Moxibustion* 2, 25–28.

Zhang, H., Zhang, Z.X. and Wu, D.Z. (1985b) Acupuncture on the unit discharge of cerebral cortex and bladder function. *Shanghai J. Acupunct. Moxibustion* 4, 28–31.

Zhang, Z.X., Zhang, H. and Wu, D.Z. (1987) Effect of acupuncture on points micturation center and related function of urinary bladder. *Acupunct. Res.* 2, 116–122.

Zhang, J.Z. and Jin, X.Y. (1995) Urethral syndrome. *Foreign Med. Sci. (Urol. Nephrol.)* 15(2), 84–86.

Zheng, H.T., Wang, S.Y., Huang, C., et al. (1996) Tonic kidney and warm yang by Acupuncture to treat urethral syndrome of women. *Shanghai J. Tradit. Chin. Med.* 11, 28.

Zhou, R.X. (1996) *Bladder Surgery.* People's medical publishing house, Beijing, pp. 15–18, 33–36.

Chapter 12

Acupuncture for Quitting Smoking

Abstract

Acupuncture treatment has certainly originated from China, yet the earliest documentary report about the use of acupuncture for quitting smoking came from the United States. Sacks L., in the US, presented the earliest report on ear needling for quitting smoking in 1975 in the *American Journal of Acupuncture* (Sacks, 1975). The acupoint chosen was the so-called "sweet taste point" or "sweet honey" point, discovered accidentally by another American James S. Olms and was published later in *American Journal of Acupuncture* (Olms, 1981). Coincidently, early practice on acupuncture for quitting smoking in China also started about the same time when the Chinese Medicine practitioners used ear acupuncture together with GV 20 for quitting smoking. The treatment course lasted one week, and after treatment for 1–3 weeks, out of 210 cases of smokers, 191 cases succeeded in quitting smoking (Wu, 1980). Since then acupuncture for quitting smoking commonly used ear acupoints as the major area of application to be supplemented with body points. Other simple techniques like ear points pressing, ear point needle embedding, etc. have also been tried. In this chapter, quitting smoking with acupuncture and psychological problems related to quitting smoking are reported.

Keywords: Quitting Smoking; Tobacco Addiction; Psychological Adherence.

12.1 Quitting Smoking with Acupuncture

Clinical reports of acupuncture to quit smoking are mainly on puncturing Auricular. The common ear acupoints used included: *Shenmen*, Mouth, Lung, Stomach, Trachea, Sympathetic Nerve, Subcortex, Endocrine, etc., while use of others such as Liver, Kidney, Spleen and Bronchus, Ear Apex, etc. were reported at a lower frequency. Usually 3–4 points were selected, each time with two ears in alternate use. The methods used included repeated mainly ear point pressing via small hard vaccaria seeds, or green beans, or in recent years, magnetic beads. Short needle direct acupuncture on the ear points was also done.

Body acupuncture was also used for quitting smoking. Outside China, the "sweet taste" acupoint was popular. The positioning of this point lied about the one thumb breadth away from the edge of the anatomical snuff-box, LU 7. Allegedly puncturing this point initiated some smokers to feel sleepy, relaxed and experience a queer sweet taste. James S. Olms (1981) who advocated this point reported in 1981 that he used he was able to make 80% of 5000 tobacco craving people quit smoking. In 1984 he reported a total effective rate was more than 90% for 2282 smokers when using this point together with ear needling and nose needling using laser (Olms, 1984). Olms also tried needling all points on the wrist along with the lung meridian of Hand-*Taiyin* and Large Intestine meridian of Hand-Yangming, but results were disappointing. Other clinical reports claimed that for the left-handers' the successful rate was lower than right-handers' (Tan, 1996).

Body needling alone had been tried, either simple manipulations or with Electro-Acupuncture (EA). For example, there was a report using LI 20, LI 11, LI 4 or ST 4, ST 36, LR 3, together with EA. A series of ten treatments gave an effective rate of 100% (Lu, 1996). The use of body needling plus EA (LI 20, LU 7, LU 6) and hot cupping (BL 13, BL 21) have been repeated to give good results. A course of five treatments completely cut out smoking in 42 patients, an effective rate of 85%, while the total effective rate reached 68.57% (Li *et al.*, 2000).

12.2 The Effective Rate of Acupuncture on Quitting Smoking

At present, there are great differences on the reports of the effective rate and quitting rate when acupuncture was used for quitting smoking. A retrospective analysis of reports showed that the lowest effective rate on completion of treatment was 43.48%. One month after completion, it dropped to 29.27%. The highest effective rate at the end of treatment was 100%, and after three months, the rate remained 100%. But one year later it dropped to 90.9%. For those who really quit at the end of treatment, the lowest rate is 8.9%, and three months later it dropped to 3.2%. The highest quitting rate three months after treatment was 100%; one year later it dropped to

72.7% (Cui and Jiang,1993). The different results could be related to the selection of acupoints, and treatment method. It could also be related to the different evaluation methods. There is one review summarizing 30 studies related to the use of acupuncture for quitting smoking. Eleven of the studies did not have a control group. It was found that only two studies showed that acupuncture was better than the placebo group, while nine studies did not review any significant difference between the two groups of treatment. Three other studies actually reported that the control group treatment effect was better than acupuncture group (Cui and Jiang, 1992).

12.3 Psychological Problems Related to Smoking and Efforts to Quit

A study was done on two groups of patients. The first group had intention to quit smoking while the second was given acupuncture for the prevention of chronic respiratory disease. The same acupoints were used for both groups. The results were as follows (Fang *et al.*, 1983):

(1) The early effective rate for those did not intended to quit was 70%, while late effective rate was 39%, suggesting that the ear acupuncture produced genuine effects, and the early results were better than late ones.

(2) For the active smokers, the early effective rate was 87%, and late rate was 71%. There was no significant difference in terms of early results between those intending to quit or not intending to quit groups. However the intend to quit group did better in the long term.

(3) Those receiving ear acupuncture claimed that during treatment, smoking failed to retain the usual "taste".

(4) Ear needling could give the fringe benefits of relieving the smokers' chronic cough and respiratory symptoms.

One study was conducted to observe the effects of psychological care in addition to ear acupoints tape-press for the treatment of smoking. Sixty cases of smoking quitters were randomly divided into a simple ear points tape-press group, and ear points tape-press plus psychological care group. For the psychological care group, as soon as there was positive responses psychological counseling was given. The results showed that ear points tape-press plus psychological care group achieved a total effective rate of 93.73%, significantly better than the simple ear points tape-press group (Sun, 2000).

12.4 Comparison between Acupuncture Treatment and Other Treatment Methods

(1) To compare the treatment effect of acupuncture and that of nicotine chewing gum on quitting smoking, Clavel conducted an experiment in which he divided 651 cases of smokers randomly into needling group (GB 8, Back of the Ball), nicotine chewing gum group, and control group. In a month, they received three treatment sessions, each for one hour. The result were as follows: the respective quitting rates of the three groups were needling group 19%, nicotine chewing gum group 22%, and control group 8%. The quitting rate of the two treatment groups were significantly better than the control group, while there was no significant difference between the two treatment groups (Clavel *et al.*, 1985). The author later also observed in another clinical research on 996 cases of smokers for quitting smoking, in which after applying the above-mentioned method for treatment for one month, the quitting rates of needling group and its placebo group, nicotine chewing gum group and its placebo group were 22%, 23%, 26% and 19% respectively. The results indicated that there was no significant difference in terms of treatment effect between treatment groups, needling group and needling placebo group (Clavel *et al.*, 1990).

(2) To compare the treatment effects on quitting smoking using acupuncture and behavioral therapy, Cottraux conducted an experiment in which 558 cases of smokers were randomly divided into the needling group (140 cases), behavioral therapy group (138 cases, using anxiety relief and self-control method), placebo medicine group (140 cases) and no treatment (140). During the 12-month follow-up visit after treatment was completed, it was found that between the needling group's quitting rate (16%), and placebo group (14%), there was no significant difference. These were better than the behavioral therapy group (7%) and no treatment group (6%) (Cottraux *et al.*, 1983).

12.5 Additional Views

Toxic effects of tobacco addiction affect not only the respiratory system and induced cancer development, but are also widely expressed in the other vital systems like musculoskeletal units and gastrointestinal tract. Addiction to smoking has a complicated background involving physiological, social and psychological issues. Standard means to help removing the harmful habit include the use of nicotine substitute, and psychological counseling. While these methods do achieve reasonable and positive results, the problem, however, remains because of recurrences. It is not uncommon to encounter cases of repeated treatments that failed to achieve the expectation. While no single method could claim supremacy, methods that are apparently yet deficient of scientific basis should still deserve fair attention.

Acupuncture as an option to induce smoking quitting may belong to the category of "unscientific" methodology. Conventional bodily puncture could be the standard choice. Ear acupuncture is becoming more and more popular because of the relative simplicity and possibility of involving the patient himself to execute self-administration of either simple puncture or acupressure (which is even more straightforward).

Using acupuncture to remove the smoking habit is not a classical methodology. It has developed out of need, probably because more conventional means are disappointing. Up to now, even within the circle of acupuncture practitioners, it is not yet widely accepted. According to the impression of the acupuncturists, one could safely assume that acupuncturing should have no direct effects on the immediate psychological adherence to tobacco smoking, since the exact physiological mechanisms leading to the addiction have remained incomplete. If acupuncture is going to help with the quitting of smoking, the mechanism could possibly be directing towards the direction and the control of the adverse effects following stopping smoking. Symptoms like nausea, chest discomfort, dizziness, thirstiness, inability to concentrate, etc. are intolerable to chronic smokers. If these symptoms could be alleviated through simple measures like acupuncture, it could be a good support to those who are determined to quit smoking and yet become miserable because of the early adverse effects. Improvement of the adverse symptoms would naturally help the patients to maintain their determination and resilience. Since adverse symptoms are either related to gastrointestinal or neurophysiological discomforts, the choice of acupoints are selected accordingly. The popular points include: *Na-guan* (內關 PC6), *Da-ling* (大陵 PC7), *Shen-men* (神門 HT7), *Shen-ting* (神庭 DU24), *Bai-hui* (百會 DU20), *He-gu* (合谷 LI4), *Tai-chong* (太沖 LR3), *Na-ting* (內庭 ST44), *Zu-san-li* (足三里 ST36), etc. For ear acupuncture, those acupuncture points related to gastrointestinal and neurophysiological effects are chosen.

Looking though available clinical reports related to acupuncture and smoking and subjecting them to a logical analysis could be contributory. However, the reviews so far have remained controversial. The authors would like to quote two clinical studies done in Hong Kong. The first one was completed in comparing the effects of the use of psychological counseling with or without the supplement of nicotine supplement (Report 1, 2009). The results showed positive results with the combined treatment but no conclusion could be made because of the lack of biostatistical evidence (Report 1, 2009; Report 2, 2009; Lam, 2005). In another study, ear acupuncture was used as a means to help quitting smoking. It is a well-planned, randomized placebo control study using sham acupoints on the ear. The results appear rather similar to the nicotine study in that both groups showed positive results, but the difference does not reach biostatistical significance. When the quality of life issue is assessed, there is clear improvement on both groups (Wing *et al.*, 2010). This latter study is designed for the cooperation of the acupuncturist and the recipients, who are encouraged to administer finger pressure on the acupoints selected to maintain an intermittent, yet continuous influence. For a bizarre neurophysiological event like addiction, active participation with enthusiasm will be essential for the expected effects. This might be important for the selection of acupuncture as a treatment option. An enthusiastic acceptance of the puncturing procedures should have positive effects on the short term and long term outcome.

References

Clavel, F., Benhamou, S., Company-Huertas, A., *et al.* (1985) Helping people to stop smoking: randomised comparison of groups being treated with acupuncture and nicotine gum with control group. *Br. Med. J.* **291**(6508), 1538–1539.

Clavel, F. and Paoletti, C. (1990) A study of various smoking cessation programs based on close to 1000 volunteers recruited from the general population: 1-month results. *Rev Epidemiol Sante Publique.* **38**(2), 133–138.

Cottraux, J.A., Harf, R., Boissel, J.P., *et al.* (1983) Smoking cessation with behaviour therapy of acupuncture — a controlled study. *Behav. Res. Ther.* **21**(4), 417–424.

Cui, M. and Jiang, A.P. (1993) Efficacy analysis of acupuncture for quitting smoking. *J. Tradit. Chin. Med.* **34**(4), 243–246.

Cui, M. and Jiang, A.P. (1992) The impact of psychological factors on the efficacy of acupuncture to quit smoking. *Shanghai J. Acupunc. Moxibustion* **4**, 33–36.

Fang, Y.A., Hou, Y.Z., Bao, G.Q., *et al.* (1983) Clinical study of auricular acupuncture to quit smoking. *Shanghai J. Acupunc. Moxibustion* **2**, 30–31.

Lam, T.H., Abdullah, A.S., Chan, S.S. and Hedley, A.J. (2005) Adherence to nicotine replacement therapy versus quitting smoking among Chinese smokers: A preliminary investigation. *Psychopharmacology* **177**(4), 400–408.

Lu, J. (1996) Clinical observation on 42 cases of quitting smoking by acupuncture. *J. Clin. Acupunc. Moxibustion* **12**(2), 22.

Li, F.L., Hao, X.L., Bian, P., *et al.* (2000) 35 cases of quitting smoking by acupuncture and cupping. *ACTA Chin. Med. Pharmacol.* **3**, 54.

Olms, J.S. (1981) How to stop smoking: Effective new acupuncture point discovered. *Am. J. Acupunc.* **9**(3), 257–260.

Report 1. (2009) A New Smoking Cessation Health Centre in Hong Kong. First interim report on the characteristics of clients attending the Smoking Cessation Health Centre (SCHC). www.smokefree.hk/cosh/ccs/file_download.xml?lang¼en&fldrid¼170. Accessed January 2009.

Report 2. (2009) Impact of smoking cessation services on smokers in Hong Kong and predictors of successful quitting. www.smokefree.hk/cosh/ccs/file_download.xml?lang¼en&fldrid¼170. Accessed January 2009.

Sacks, L. (1975) Drug addiction, alcoholism, smoking, obesity treated by auricular staplepuncture. *Am. J. Acupunc.* **3**, 147–150.

Sun, C.X. (2000) Roles of psychological nursing played in the course of auricle point applying to help individuals giving up smoking. *Shangxi Nursing J.* **14**(2), 69.

Tan, X.H. (1996) Positioning identification of Tian Mei — a new acupoint for quitting smoking. *Chin Acupunc. Moxibustion* **12**, 51.

Wu, Y.R. (1980) Acupuncture for quitting smoking efficacy analysis of 210 cases. *J. Tradit. Chin. Med.* **5**, 48–49.

Yun-Kwok, W., Anna, L., Eliza, L.Y., *et al.* (2010) Auricular acupressure for smoking cessation: a pilot randomized controlled trial. *Med. Acupunc.* **22**(4), 265–271.

Chapter 13

Acupuncture for Other Conditions — Obesity, Skin Conditions, Hyperthyroidism and Ulcerative Colitis

Abstract

Many clinical problems, in spite of repeated attempts on treatment remain disturbing. The application of complementary treatment is often the result of patients' disappointment and clinicians' enthusiasm to help. Acupuncture is an important component of Traditional Chinese Medicine. The concept of acupuncture is based on an assumption of maintaining an internal balance through the stimulation of special points along the meridians. Acupuncture, therefore, enjoys a free utilization as a harmonizing procedure. When modern practitioners start to utilize acupuncture as alternative means of treatment, their scientific medicine background is influencing them to take a specific approach for the treatment of specific pathologies. Unlike acupuncture experts, they ignore the general concept of bringing harmony to physiological imbalance. Once they are convinced they apply the traditional technique to areas of popular concern like obesity, and skin conditions affecting cosmesis, and difficult situation occurring in endocrine and autoimmune diseases like thyrotoxicosis and ulcerative colitis.

This chapter has no intention of making a comprehensive review on the new areas of application of acupuncture, but would attempt to give some discussion on examples of the current popular uses.

Keywords: Cancer; Obesity; Autoimmune Diseases; Skin Conditions; Hyperthyroidism; Ulcerative Colitis.

13.1 Acupuncture and Obesity

The literature review showed that acupuncture for weight reduction has been widely used, and clinical research has been plentiful. Controversies exist in the following areas:

(1) Acupoint selection: In traditional acupuncture documents, there have never been specialized descriptions related to obesity. Current selections, such as the so-called "Obesity Three Points" (Tang *et al.*, 2004) (i.e. CV 12, GB 26 and ST 36); *Hua Tuo*'s paravertebral points (Shen *et al.*, 2000); the eight points around the umbilicus (Cheng *et al.*, 2007) (CV 9, CV 7, ST 26 (bilateral), ST 25 (bilateral), ST 24 (bilateral)), etc. are all related to experts' personal interests. It could be found that the most popular weight loss points used are ST 36, ST 25, SP 6, CV 12 and ST 40, when gastrointestinal repletion was diagnosed. LI 11, LI 4, ST 37, ST 44 were added, for "spleen vacuity" and "damp obstruction" SP 9 was added, for liver depression and "*qi* stagnation". BL 18, LR 3 and CV 6 were added, for heart-liver vacuity. BL 15, BL 20, PC 6 and HT 7 were added, for spleen-kidney yang vacuity or KI 3, KI 7, GV 4, BL 20 and BL 23 were added (Xu *et al.*, 2004).

(2) Treatment methods varied. Many different methods of acupuncture treatment for simple obesity have been documented reports, such as body needling, EA, moxibustion, ear points (including magnetic and pressure taping), head needling, warm needling, elongated needle, catgut embedding, fire cupping, etc. Controversies had been multiple. However, the general feeling is that a combination of many methods might give better results.

(3) Acupuncture experts also took reference to traditional Chinese Medicine concepts of diagnosis as helpful guidelines to the choice of acupoints and method of administration. The results were claimed to be better (Wei *et al.*, 2002; Mi, 2005; Li and Liu, 1998).

13.2 Additional Views

Obesity is a physiological problem. Obesity is also a socio-psychological problem. To start with, the definition of obesity could be controversial. The standard body weight could be defined as a function relevant to body weight and height. However, even those defined as the "standard" body weight might either personally feel or considered to be "obese". As the general public is constantly influenced by advertising efforts in the commercial community when beauty is advocated to be indispensably related with slimness, the meaning of "obesity" is therefore further confused. Whoever is not slim might incorrectly be considered "obese".

Currently, preventing obesity and keeping slim has become a fashion in the affluent society. Hence, means to keep slim has commercial value and enterprises provoking the pursuit of slimness have flourished. Multiple means are being used to achieve the control of obesity or pushing further, to attain slimness, and bodily contour beauty.

When we discuss about obesity and the related treatment, we must bear in mind the complexity of the problem and the effects of commercialization. Acupuncture has never been documented as a treatment means for obesity *per se*. When treatment of obesity fails to reach clients' expectation, acupuncture comes into the consideration of enthusiasts. In response to the clients' need, acupuncture experts start an active practice of obesity treatment.

Acupuncturists need to assume that excess weight is a manifestation of imbalance between yin and yang, and therefore treatment policy has to be developed according to the observation of the nature of the imbalance: whether it is due to deficient *qi* (形盛气虚) or excessive phlegm (肥人多痰); whether it is secondarily due to deficiency or excessiveness of the "spleen" function. Acupuncturists therefore tend to adopt a dynamic policy, altering the acupoints according to the changing observations. The parameters are not confined to body weight itself, but other manifestations like bodily strength, physical resilience, are also important targets of assessment.

The selection of acupuncture points include those known to strengthen "*qi*" and "spleen" and those to remove moisture and phlegm. Those points are related to meridian of "stomach" and "spleen", including *Tian-Shu* (天枢, ST25), *Zu-san-li* (足三里, ST36), *Xia-ju-xu* (下巨虚 ST39), *Feng-long* (丰隆, ST40), *Da-heng* (大横, SP15), *San-yin-jiao* (三阴交 SP6), *Yin-ling-quan* (阴陵泉 SP9), etc. Sometimes other acupuncture points used for diuresis are also used. These include *Shen-yu* (肾俞 BL 23), *Qi-hai* (气海 RN6), *Guan-yuan* (关元 RN4), etc. When it is observed that if the diagnosis is related to gastrointestinal "heat", stagnation of "*qi*" and "liver" function, other acupuncture points could be considered, like *He-gu* (合谷 LI4), *Tai-chong* (太冲 LR3), *Qi-men* (期门 LR14), and *Yang-ling-quan* (阳陵泉 GB34). Among the obese, clinical symptoms might include those of neurasthenia. Under such circumstance, acupoints indicated for psychological stabilization can be used. These acupuncture points include *Shen-men* (神门 HT7), *Na-guan* (内关 PC6), *Da-ling* (大陵 PC7), etc.

The complexities of acupuncture choices have well indicated that obesity is never simple and straightforward. The policy for treatment needs dynamic adjustment in response to changing clinical behaviour and detection of additional clinical signs requires an appropriate adjustment of treatment. Not only is modification of acupuncture points necessary, but the choice between manual and electrical technique needs to be considered as well, and whether moxibustion could be beneficial needs special considerations.

Looking through current literature, other divergent views about the choice of acupuncture points and puncturing techniques are available. Some experts even advocate the routine use of alternate choices of acupoint groups, changing meridians and changing techniques.

Electro-Acupuncture (EA) has been very much advocated. Acupoints chosen include CV 12, ST 21, ST 24, ST 25, SP 15, SP 14 and CV 5 (Ren, 2007).

Others used BL 20, BL 21, BL 22, ST 25, ST 28, CV 9, CV 12, CV 6, SP 15, ST 36, ST 40, GB 34 and SP 6 (Li and Deng, 2004).

Moxibustion is also popular, using the same acupoints (Tang and Li, 1992).

Ear acupuncture or acupressure has been used widely because it requires active participation of the patients themselves. The major ear-points used are endocrine, subcortex, spleen, mouth, adrenal, abdomen and lung (Jiang and Zhang, 1997; Lu, 1986; Peng, 2005).

Catgut embedding at the selected acupoints have been used to acquire long-term continuous effects. The acupoints used are CV 12, ST 25, CV 6 and ST 37 (Zhang and Fu, 2006; Wang, 2006).

We believe that acupuncture for obesity will probably never be adopted as the standard treatment, because of its deficient historical application and deficient physiological evidences. Nevertheless, in view of the generally lack of satisfaction among overweight people seeking treatment, acupuncture as an alternative option could be well-supported.

Advocates of allopathic medicine should not be overly skeptical about the application of acupuncture as a means to treat obesity. Modern clinics in obesity management have been applying new but immature principles on the treatment of obesity. The new but immature principles include the assumption that obesity is due to "subclinical toxicities" related to the consumption of a variety of unhealthy food items. Alternatively, assumingly the lack of control of bodily fat could also be the result of deficiency or excessiveness of some internal hormonal secretion. These clinics are starting to identify special measurable chemical and hormonal parameters for the identification of the cause of obesity with the intension of subsequent management.

When one takes a critical look at this new approach to obesity management, one realizes that the alleged evidences are yet short of convincing support. A loss of balance between internal secretions of opposing functions could be interpreted as a state of loss of internal harmony. The new clinics for the management of obesity, therefore, are apparently in agreement with the use of acupuncture, which works towards the maintenance of the internal balance and physiological harmony.

13.3 Acupuncture for Skin Conditions

13.3.1 *Acne*

Common acne is a skin disease commonly found among adolescent youth. This condition tends to gradually abate, but a few patients are continuously bothered by the unsightly ailment. Affliction is mostly on the face; in the process of development it might get infected, hence making the skin rough and unsightly. Acne is related to excessive adolescent hormonal secretion, closely related to endocrine function, and dietary habits.

In traditional Chinese Medicine theory acne is a manifestation of internal imbalance, closely related to the lung, spleen and liver. As "lung governs the skin and body hair", impaired lung *qi* is responsible for acne. "Spleen governs the flesh" means spleen-stomach damp-heat lies on the skin, and contributes towards acne. Irritating foods that are sweet, pungent, sour and hot, generate heat, thus leading to spleen-stomach damp-heat. Similarly cigarette smoking and alcohol contribute towards the formation of acne.

The following acupuncture techniques have been applied:

(1) Body acupuncture: Acupuncture points used include: LI 11, LI 4, CV 12, ST 25, CV 6, ST 36, LR 3 and SP 6 (Wang, 2004).

(2) Acupoint injection: Acupuncture points used include: BL 13, BL 25, EX-CA 1, BL 18, BL 20 and BL 21 (Cheng and Ma, 1999).

(3) Ear points acupuncture: Using bilat lung, liver, endocrine, subcortex, with or without body acupuncture (Zhong and Qiu *et al.*, 2001).

(4) Moxibustion: 2–3 acupuncture points like those selected for body punctures are chosen for moxibustion (Ye and Li, 1996).

(5) Pricking and cupping: The popular acupoint used is GV 14, which is pricked with a three-edged needle until bleeding appears, after which cupping is applied (Ma and Bao *et al.*, 1994; Huang and Huang, 1999; Cao Weimin, 1995).

13.3.2 *Yellow-brown macules*

Yellow-brown macules, nicknamed pregnancy spots and butterfly spots, appear on the face as local symmetrical butterfly shaped, light brown or brownish pigmentations. They most often appear on the nose, forehead, zygomatic region, around the mouth and cheek. Minor skin injuries often turn into such macules. The surface of the lesion is smooth, without scale, and when exposed to sunlight the pigment becomes further darkened. Yellow-brown macules could also be related to some chronic diseases, endocrine, disturbances, ultraviolet light, and certain drugs. For female patients the macules could also be related to pregnancy, oral contraceptives and cosmetics (Aoyang and Yang, 2003). Excessive black pigments in the subcutaneous cells are the core pathology (Yu, 1994).

Theories of disharmony, insufficiency of the liver and kidney, dietary irregularity, splenic problems, and dual depletion of *qi* and blood leading to *qi* stagnation and blood stasis. Modern medicine aims at supportive treatment or local application of pigment elimination, and there are also reports of laser treatment. Acupuncture treatment might be an option.

(1) Body acupuncture: The major points used are GV 23 and GB 14; major points at the nose is Hall of Impression and LI 20; at zygomatic region, the major points are SI 8 and ST 2; at the cheek, the major point is ST 6; around the mouth, the major points are GV 26, LI 19, ST 4 and CV

24; at *ashi* point (needling mostly aims at darker brown area). For distal point selection, the common ones are ST 36, SP 6, LI 4 and LR 3, or related transport points at the back, abdomen alarm points and selected matching point from pattern differentiation (Qian, 1992).

(2) Acu-point injection: Acupoints used are BL 13, BL 15, BL 18, BL 20 and BL 23 (Zhang, 1996).

(3) Ear point acupuncture: The major points selected were endocrine and *Shenmen*. This could also be combined with bloodletting (Wang and Ma, 1996). Likewise, pricking and bloodletting can be combined (Li and Zhao, 1992).

Points selected on the face include GB 14, ST 6, ST 2, Hall of Impression and LI 20 (Zhang *et al.*, 2004).

13.3.3 *Warts*

Warts are a benign epidermal new growth caused by the vacuoles nipple polyma virus. There are four types: common wart, flat wart, plantar wart, and pointed wart. It starts as a pin-head size, then pea size. At the initial affliction, there is usually just a single wart, then the viral lesion spreads centrifugally outwards to several or dozens. Usually there are no obvious symptoms, but occasionally it hurts when pressed, and easily bleeds when it is rubbed or hit. Warts usually attack fingers, feet, and nail margins, though morbidity is slow and often it heals by itself.

(1) Acupuncture: Needling treatment is as follows: A 3 cm long acupuncture needle is inserted into the mother wart centre, deep down to its root, then it is withdrawn to subcutaneous level. This is repeated several times with perpendicular insertion. After that, insertion was repeated 4–5 times on surrounding direction of the wart, and this is counted as one treatment. When the needle was withdrawn, the tip would not leave from the skin, and for every insertion the needle tip must reach the root of the wart. There should be some loose feeling under the needle, and after a break of 15 days, the second treatment is applied. After the second treatment, there would be 20 days interval before the third treatment is carried out (Dai and Lu, 2007).

Alternately, applying acupuncture to *ashi* point is another way to treat common wart. First routine sterilization was carried out on the affected local skin, two 0.5 cun filiform needles were directly inserted into the common wart centre and edge respectively (meeting point of wart and skin), using twirling-turning manipulation to a depth of 0.1–0.4 cun (depending on the how deep the wart root is), needles retained for 30–40 min, and in between there were 2–3 manipulations. After one needling, there should be an interval of 15–20 days, and those who are not healed would have a second needling (Qiu Yurui, 1994).

(2) Plum-Blossom Needle: The plum-blossom needling method is applied to treat the wart over the "mother area". Then bigger sizes are treated. After local sterilization, the wart is heavily tapped with plum-blossom needle 5–10 times, producing congestion and exudations (Wang *et al.*, 1997; Liu, 1994).

13.4 Acupuncture for Hyperthyroidism

Hyperthyroidism refers to a high functional state of the thyroid gland due to increased secretion of the thyroid gland hormone, leading to a rise in the activities of various physiological systems. The typical manifestation is fatigue, even after normal activities, intolerance to heat with hyperhidrosis, palpitations, and weight loss in spite of excessive eating. Hyperthyrotoxic patients are also dysphoric and irritable, and sleeping poorly. Physical signs include hand tremor, myasthenia, increased heart rate, and for females, dysmenorrhea or amenorrhea. Some patients develop different degrees of exophthalmos. The laboratory findings include increased levels of serum T4, T3, FT3, FT4, the thyroid uptake rate of ^{131}I is also increased, while TSH level is lowered. Hyperthyroidism could happen in any age, though more frequently found in the middle and young females. The standard medications include anti-thyroid hormone therapy and ancillary drug treatment. Radioactive iodine treatment and surgery operation to remove the over-active thyroid are other options (Sun *et al.*, 2003). Standard treatment is most of the time effective. Acupuncture treatment may be considered as an additional ancillary treatment when unsatisfactory results are presented.

13.4.1 *Summary and discussion*

A great deal of clinical applications and research reports are available in China in the recent decades. Basically a set of treatment programs has been formulated, and there has been more systemic research on various factors that influence acupuncture treatment outcomes. Treatment primarily aims at boosting yin and clearing fire, and by means of freeing liver and discharging heat, transforming phlegm and moving stasis to a more balanced activity. As for acu-points selection, the major points include ST 10, "Upper Celestial Pillar, "*Qi* Goitre", ST 36, SP 6, PC 6 and PC 5.

Factors which affect acupuncture effect mainly appear in the following aspects: (1) the morbid condition itself: the extent of thyromegaly, whether or not accompanied with exophthalmos, the extent of changes of biochemical indices; (2) relationship between treatment course and treatment effect: the effective rate of three treatment courses is significantly higher than that of one; (3) relationship between treatment time and relapse rate: those who receive only one treatment face a higher rate of relapse, while those with more than two continuous treatment courses tend to relapse less; and (4) relationship between duration of morbidity and treatment time: initial attacks respond much better to treatment than late cases.

Acupuncturists' views on hyperthyroidism carry a strong emphasis on a control of excessive "internal heat". The symptoms of irritability, palpitation, insomnia, hyperactivities, etc. are manifestations of "excessive heat". In the viewpoint of Chinese Medicine practitioners, "internal heat" could be related to "liver", "heart", and "stomach". Of the different systems "heart" is considered the most important, so harmonizing the internal heat of the heart system would induce secondary positive effects on the other systems.

With this background knowledge, acupuncturists have chosen four acupuncture points, viz. *Na-guan* (内关 PC6), *Jian-shi* (间使 PC5), *Zu-san-li* (足三里 ST36), and *San-yin-jian* (三阴交 SP6) as leading choices for acupuncture treatment for hyperthyroidism. Of the four acupuncture points, *Nei-guan* and *Jian-shi* are well known to down-tune excessive "heart" activities. This view of the acupuncturists is well supported in the classical teaching of the medical classics, under sections of the "Balance of the five forces" (Huangdi Neijing, 2010).

Some acupuncturists use heart rate and rhythm as guiding signs to the choice of acupuncture treatment and assessment of treatment results. They have also advocated an analysis of the other parameters of thyroid function as additional measures to adjust treatment. Observations are also made on the other symptoms like weakness, hyperhyosis, weight loss and bowel activities. According to classical teaching, such symptoms are indicators of deficiencies of "*qi*" and "*yin*", which could be accordingly managed. The choice of *Zu-san-li* and *San-yin-jian* are all directed towards the strengthening of *qi* and *yin*.

Hence the choice of the four acupuncture points is a clever, pragmatic practice, capable of utilizing the classical theories to solve clinical problems.

When hyperthyroidism is complicated with glandular hypertrophy or exothalmus, local acupuncture options become important considerations. The choice of appropriate acupuncture points in the head and neck regions is important. Moreover, the direction of puncture, angulation, depth and manipulation would also need special consideration. *Feng-chi* (风池 GB20) and *Shang-tian-chi* (上天池) are two popular points to be chosen for exothalmus.

Lastly, acupuncturists commonly use combined treatment, i.e. while acupuncture is being performed in parallel while anti-hyperthyroid pharmaceuticals are administered, particularly when complications like exophthalmia coexist. Acupuncturists believe that acupuncture is particularly valuable, when adverse drug effects occur or when over-lengthy administration of pharmaceuticals produce unusual problems. After all there has been no study proving that acupuncture could replace the standard forms of therapy. On the contrary, many reports used acupuncture as a supplement, in addition to standard treatment, and reported good results.

In the standard hospital practice, hyperthyroidism enjoys a standard treatment after proper diagnosis. The established regime of drug treatment, with radioisotope therapy and rarely surgical intervention for more resistant cases, is considered standard. The standard regime usually gives highly satisfactory results and, unless administered too untimely, adverse effects and complications do not often appear. The use of acupuncture to supplement the standard treatment regime deserves special consideration when drug adversity and other complications occur. Endocrinologists should bear in mind the availability of the traditional practice that could supplement their modern treatment.

13.5 Acupuncture and Ulcerative Colitis

In 1875, Wilks and Moxon first offered a description of this condition, taking it out from category of chronic diarrhea to become an independent disease. To differentiate it from other inflammatory condition of the colon, it is called "non-specific ulcerative colon inflammation".

Ulcerative colitis (UC) is a disease with unknown exact etiology. The chronic inflammatory affection mainly occurs in the colon mucous membrane, producing ulcerative erosions, mostly occurring towards the end of the colon, but it could spread proximally and distally. The major symptoms are bloody mucous stool, abdominal pain, tenesmus, and diarrhea. There is a great difference between its mild and severe form. The course of illness is mostly slow with recurrent tendencies of acute fulminating presentations. There are many theories on the etiology of this disease; the major one maintains that it is related to the following factors: infection, psychological factor, hereditary and local factors within the large intestine (enzymes, sensitivities, disturbed immunological defense mechanisms). The patient's body has significant increase of IgM, IgG, IgA increases in lymphocyte exchange rate, T cells, B cells, etc. (Zheng *et al.*, 1993).

Owing to the uncertainty of the disease etiology and pathogenesis, and clinical manifestation complexity with many complications, up to now medical treatment could only offer merely symptomatic relief, and not full recovery from the disease. Symptomatic relief is provided through the use of antibiotics, glucocorticoids and corticotrophins, and immunosuppressants. Surgical treatment is considered a last option. Acupuncture and moxibustion have been tried after the obvious reason of disappointing results with conventional treatment.

13.5.1 *Summary and discussion*

Taking the general view of recent studies on the use of acupuncture for ulcerative collitis, the following observations could be recorded:

(1) The effects of acupuncture on the symptom control of UC is clear, especially when applied in the early phase of treatment.

(2) In the clinical application, it is mostly a combination of needling and moxibustion or moxibustion and medicines, that give the best response. The application of acupuncture alone is not as effective.

(3) Acupoint characteristics: Acupoints selected are mainly based on several points in the lower abdomen on CV, stomach, large intestine meridians along their lower uniting point and alarm point, such as CV 8, CV 6, CV 4,CV 12 (stomach meridian alarm point) on CV, stomach meridian uniting point ST 36, large intestine alarm point ST 25, large intestine lower uniting point ST 37. The treatment principles and acupuncture points selected follow the Chinese Medicine guidelines on "diarrhea" and "dysentery".

Ulcerative colitis and its related Crohn's disease are rare pathological conditions affecting the endothelial layer of the bowel. There could be a high frequency of familial tendency, and the nature of the inflammatory changes could be an autoimmune process. While they are treated like other autoimmune conditions, where either special cytotoxic drugs or steroids could be useful, treatment outcome is often unpredictable. The ulcerative inflammatory processes unfortunately, tend to produce life-threatening presentations when bleeding and perforation of the guts occur. Before the disastrous events, clinicians and patients want to try every possible means to help controlling the development of exacerbations.

Acupuncture is, in fact, not an obviously suitable treatment option. Acupuncture could be useful controlling acute symptoms of diarrhea or abdominal colic; however, the bizarre nature of the inflammatory component would not be reachable by needling.

Facing this challenge of serious clinical manifestation with obscure cause, acupuncturists would apply general meridian theories in their execution of puncture treatment. Three basic states might be identifiable: "dampness", "heat", and "coolness". The most generally observed physiological state could be "dampness", which is enhanced further with the presence of blood and mucus in the diarrhea. When diarrhea suddenly stops, it is interpreted as the state of "coolness" taking over. Deficiency of the stomach and spleen is often the explanation. Treatment goes accordingly: controlling "dampness" or supplementing deficiencies. The selected acupoints therefore, are those along the stomach meridian occupying positions below the umbilicus, e.g. *Shen-que* (神阙 RN8), *Shui-fen* (水分 RN9), *Tian-shu* (天枢 ST25), *Qi-hai* (气海 RN6), *Guan-yuan* (关元 RN4), *Shang-ju-xu* (上巨虚 ST37), *Xia-ju-xu* (下巨虚 ST39), and *Zu-san-li* (足三里 ST36), etc.

When treatment does not give guaranteed results, constant repetitive measures become important. One way to achieve a sustained effect of acupuncture is to combine moxibustion with addition of a ginger patch or herbal cake placed between the abdominal skin and the moxibustion. The procedure gives a feeling of intra-abdominal warmth, which is particularly appreciated by patients suffering from bloody diarrhea. Moxibustion with ginger patch over the lower abdomen is a simple procedure that could be practiced by the patients themselves at home.

When the condition deteriorates into blood-stained stools, acupuncturists would add acupuncture points that harmonize blood and circulation by using acupoints like *Xue-hai* (血海 SP10), and *Yang-ling-quan* (阳陵泉 GB34). Preventive puncturing sessions to help balancing the deficiencies are important for a proper trial of acupuncture effects.

Whether acupuncture and moxibustion serve as symptomatic control during the attack of ulcerative colitis, or whether acupuncture and moxibustion do help the change the ulcerative inflammatory changes in the epithelium of the large bowel, remain to be explored.

References

Cao, W.M. (1995) Clinical observation of 396 cases treated by crochet needle with cupping for control of acne. Chin. Acupunct. Moxibustion **5**, 13–14.

Cheng, Q.L. and Ma, X.K. (1999) Acupoint injection and cosmetic acupuncture for the treatment of 275 cases with acne. *Shanghai J. Acupunct. Moxibustion* **8**(4), 17.

Cheng, L., Chen, M.G. and Yang, H. (2007) Influence of acupuncture on insulin resistance in simple obesity patients. *Shanghai J. Acupunct. Moxibustion* **26**(2), 8–10.

Dai, H.Y. and Lu, Y. (2007) Clinical research of acupuncture treatment for multiple common warts, plantar warts in 126 cases. *China Modern Doctor* **45**(5), 65.

Huang, B.Y. and Huang, J.B. (1999) The plum-blossom needle and cupping methods for the treatment of acne in 100 cases. *J. Fujian Coll. Tradit. Chin. Med.* **9**(4), 26.

Huangdi, N. (2010) Ancient Chinese Medicine Press.

Jiang, Y. and Zhang, Q.P. (1997) Auricular bead treatment of simple obesity. *Clin. J. Anhui Tradit. Chin. Med.* **9**(1), 55.

Li, L.S. and Zhao ZB. (1992) Clinical observation of pricking and cupping and the Auricular acupressure for facial chloasma of 486 cases. *Chin. Acupunct. Moxibustion* **12**(6), 7–8.

Liu, J.L. (1994) Fire-needle treatment of *verruca plana*. *J. Clin. Acupunct. Moxibustion* **10**(6), 29.

Li, J. and Liu, Z.C., (1998) Clinical observation of 40 cases of simple obesity treated with acupuncture. *Chin. Acupunct. Moxibustion* **18**(9), 539.

Li, J.M. and Deng, Y.J. (2004) Efficacy observation of 93 cases with simple obesity treated with electro-acupuncture. *Clin. J. Tradit. Chin. Med.* **16**(5), 479.

Lu, M.Z., Zhou, K.Y., Liang. Z.Z, *et al.* (1986) 1000 cases of clinical efficacy report of auricular acupressure method to control body weight. *Guizhou Med. J.* **10**(5), 6–7.

Ma, R. and Bao, H.L. (1994) Acupoint *Dazhui* bloodletting and cupping for the treatment of acne in 102 cases. *Chin. Acupunct. Moxibustion* **5**, 46.

Mi, Y.Q. (2005) Clinical study on acupuncture for treatment of 80 cases of simple obesity. *Chin. Acupunct. Moxibustion* **25**(2), 95–98.

Ouyang, H. and Yang, Z.B. (2003) *Integrative Medicine for the Diagnosis and Treatment of Facial Skin Diseases*. People's Medical Publishing House, pp. 129–130.

Peng, J.Q. (2005) 150 cases of simple obesity treated with auricular acupressure. *Mod. Med. Health* **21**(16), 2187.

Qian, J.F. (1992) Acupuncture treatment for freckles of 30 cases. *Shanghai J. Acupunct. Moxibustion* **3**, 23.

Qiu, Y.R. (1994) A summary of 40 cases of puncturing Ashi acupoint for the treatment of *verruca vulgaris*. New J. Tradit. Chin. Med. **6**, 35.

Ren, Y.Y. (2007) Abdomen electrical needle in the treatment of simple obesity: Curative effect. Observation of 136 cases. *Modern Tradit. Chin. Med.* **27**(2), 46–47.

Sun, Y.A., Duan, W.R., Li, D.A., *et al.* (2003) *Practical Therapeutics of Endocrine and Metabolic Diseases*. People's Medical Publishing House, pp. 99–103.

Tang, C.Y. and Li, E.T. (1992) Clinical obsetration on moxibustion for weight reduction. *Acupunct. Res.* **4**, 261–262.

Tang, Q.F., Deng, Q.P. and Xu, Q.Y. (2004) 50 Cases of simple obesity treated with fat three-pin. *New J. Tradit. Chin. Med.* **36**(10), 50–51.

Wang, S.L. (2006) Clinical observation of 100 cases of obesity treated with the acupoint catgut embedding therapy. *J. Practi. Tradit. Chin. Int. Med.* **20**(1), 97.

Wang, H.T. and Ma, K. (1996) Ear bleeding for treatment of chloasma of 120 cases. *Henan Tradit. Chin. Med.* **16**(2), 51.

Wang, R.H., Zhang, G.M., Wu, H.D., *et al.* (1997) Clinical observation on acupuncture treatment of child cerebral palsy. *Chin. Acupunct. Moxibustion* **1**, 30.

Wang, H. (2004) Efficacy observation of He's three-way method for treatment of acne. *Beijing J. Tradit. Chin. Med.* **23**(4), 201–203.

Wei, Q.L. and Liu, Z.C. (2002) Comparison between auricular acupuncture, body acupuncture and combination of auricular and body acupuncture in treating simple obesity. *J. Nanjing Univ. Tradit. Chin. Med.* **18**(1), 45–47.

Xu, B., Liu, Z.C., Zhang, Z.C,, *et al.* (2004) Basic thinking and methods of establishing clinical programs for acupuncture treatment of obesity. *Chin. Acupunct. Moxibustion* **24**(2), 129–133

Ye, P.C. and Li, M.L. (1996) Ear thread embedding for the therapy of acne. *J. Clin. Acupunct. Moxibustion* **12**(12), 13.

Yu, C.Y. (1994) Changes of superoxide dismutase in different skin diseases. *Chin. J. Dermatovenereol.* **8**(3), 153–154.

Zhang, J. (1996) Drug injection in back *shu* acupoints for the treatment of 92 cases of melisma. *Beijing J. Tradit. Chin. Med.* **3**, 28–29.

Zhang, W., Lou, B.D., Long, Z.J., *et al.* (2004) The method of Wai needle hanging needling for the treatment of melasma and the influence on serum SOD and E3. *J. Chin. Physician* **32**(5), 36–37.

Zhang, Z.C. and Fu, W.B. (2006) Catgut implantation at acupoint for treatment of 30 cases of simple obesity. *Shaanxi J. Tradit. Chin. Med.* **26**(9), 1122–1124.

Zheng, Z.T., Huang, C.T. and Wang, Z.J. (1993) *Gastroenterology.* Second edition. People's Medical Publishing House, pp. 646–655.

Zhong, J.P. and Qiu, X.H. (2001) The auricular acupoint cut for the treatment of acne in 50 cases. *Clin. J. Anhui Tradit. Chin. Med.* **13**(3), 193.

Chapter 14

Discovery of Novel Acupuncture Points

Abstract

Electronic technology has been used in the course of search for objective evidences of body surface meridian locus and the transmission along the meridian. Acupuncture points have been found to have low resistance characteristics. Such characteristics were first reported by the Japanese expert, Nakatani Yoshio, in the 1950s. Thereafter, a great deal of research materials came out from China and other countries regarding skin surface electrical characteristics such as electrical resistance, conductivity, anti capacity, potential, etc. Development of relevant instruments for multiple detections followed. However, skin surface studies alone is not in line with the traditional meridian theories, which refers to multidimensional structures in accordance with different physiological and pathological states.

Keywords: Acupuncture Points; Surface Electric Potentials; Transmission Needle.

14.1 Research on Surface Electrical Characteristics of Acupuncture Points

When Nakatani Yoshio of Japan used direct current to set up a circuit on the patient's skin, he found that at certain points on the skin the conductivity is higher than the general area: he called them the good conductivity points. A line connecting all these points was called the good conductive network. Consequently it was found that these lines and points were very similar to meridians and transport points of Chinese traditional acupuncture charts (Nakatani, 1956).

Relevant research in China also confirmed the low resistance (high current) characteristics.

(1) An observational study was conducted on 25 adult volunteers and the following results were found: the ST 36 yang meridian was spread over many member zones, and was running the longest and most complicated path, while the Conception Vessel (CV) and Governor Vessel (GV) channels were spread out along the midline on the front and back of the trunk, yet within the area where different meridians merge, the surface low resistance points still move along meridians. Those points unrelated to meridians were few, and mostly occurred at the back. The low resistance points were concentrated on five areas, basically in line with GV and on the inner and outer lateral lines within the bladder meridian (Huang *et al.*, 1993). It was also found that the occurrence of low resistance points among females was significantly higher than males (Yang *et al.*, 1997).

(2) Other studies yielded different conclusions. In one, 224 normal persons were investigated for the relationship between the electrical conductivity and skin temperature. Results revealed that (i) the points on the head and face had the highest electrical conductivity and body trunk was next, the back was higher than the sacral region, the chest was higher than the abdomen, and for the limbs, proximal were higher than distal regions; (ii) concerning skin temperature, the points with high electrical conductivity also had higher temperature; and vice versa; and (iii) In a healthy person, there might not exist a "good conductivity meridian", as a "good conductivity meridian" might appear only under certain pathological conditions, which deserve further research (Zeng *et al.*, 1958a).

(3) Surface resistance, is influenced by factors like sweating, room temperature, humidity, mental state, electrode-skin interface, and design of the electrode. Studies showed:

(i) The larger the size of the electrode, the higher the electrical conductivity, and vice versa. Those acupoints with greater electrical conductivity were less affected by the electrode size.

(ii) Increase of pressure in contact with the skin would increase electrical conductivity; the influence of pressure became less significant with larger electrodes.

(iii) Using small electrodes, when the contact with the skin was set at 68 g/10 ml^2, moving up to 104 g/10 ml^2, electrical conductivity was gradually increased with the extension of energizing time. The increase of electrical conductivity value was greater, from 30 s to 120 s. A continuation led to a smaller increase.

(iv) Using large electrodes, the results were just the opposite; once the electrode touched the skin, electrical conductivity became greater, thereafter it is rapidly reduced, reaching the bottom after 30 to 40 s. It was therefore recommended that when carrying out surface electrical conductivity tests, three factors should be observed: (a) regardless of electrodes sizes, meter reading must be done within the same fixed time; (b) for large electrodes the pressure factor is not significant but for small electrodes the pressure influence must be carefully dealt with; and (c) when electrode-skin contact pressure is great, electrical conductivity might appear too high and the reverse is also true (Zeng *et al.*, 1958b). Similar findings were observed in animal experiments (Liu, 1989).

(4) The investigation of acupuncture point voltamperage characteristics is also one of the research areas acupuncture point electrical studies. Studies have found: (a) the voltamperage area (reflecting the high and low resistance) of LU 9 and LI 20 compared with the control group showed no significant difference; and (b) a normal person after blood donation, showed significant changes in the LI 20 acupuncture point voltamperage. There was no such change on LU 9. Results could have indicated that the LI 20 voltamperage could be more sensitively reflecting body *qi*-and circulatory changes (Wei *et al.*, 2003).

14.2 Detection of Surface Electrical Characteristics

To minimize the influence of outside factors on the experimental results of acupuncture point detection, researchers are trying hard to improve the method of detection of surface electrical characteristics. For example, using bipolar electrodes, the electrical characteristics between two points could be better compared. Using quadruplet electrodes the resistance of a small zone under the skin could be detected without worrying about the skin condition, humidity, pressure and detection time.

There is a device called "automatic meridian points detection system" which could rapidly detect the surface electrical data (Deng and Yin, 1998). Another device using a quadruplet electrode consisting of two groups of entirely identical electrodes on the same tiny piece of electrode plate is used to detect acupuncture point resistance, while at the same time checking the non-acupuncture point resistance (Zhang, 1995).

14.3 The Development of Transmission Needle

The research on the physical and chemical characteristics of meridians and acupuncture points has attracted many bioengineers' attention. Attempts to develop a calcium ionizing sensory transmission needle (Wang and Ren, 2002), and a thermo sensory transmission needle (Wang *et al.*, 2003), have been made. These needles might be able to monitor *in vivo* the real time and movement of calcium ions in the tissues of the acupuncture points, as well as the temperature changes, the oxygen tension and pH values (Shen *et al.*, 2004).

These sensory transmission needles have provided new thoughts on a more precise exploration of the biochemical characteristics of the meridians and the acupuncture points.

14.4 The Existing Issues on Acupuncture Point Characteristics

An overview of the research attempts of the recent five decades on acupuncture point characteristics (including voltamperage, electrical conductivity, anti-capacity and inductance, etc.), revealed a number of common observations while the research target has been concentrated on surface skin points. The so-called electrical studies have indicated that: (1) comparing with the traditional concept of acupuncture points and meridians, the electrical detections were not entirely equivalent; (2) the surface detections are affected by many physical and pathological factors, and need not be absolutely relied on; (3) electrical detections do not reflect changes in the deeper structures and do not follow the traditional concept of Chinese Medicine;

and (4) it might be suggested that during the treatment course of acupuncture, observations could be made on the dynamic changes of the electrical characteristics, which might be able to serve as assessment criteria.

References

Deng, C.L. and Yin, K.J. (1998) *Experimental Acupuncture Science.* People's Medical Publishing House, pp. 201.

Huang, X.Q., Xu, J.S. and Wu, H.B. (1993) Observation on the Distribution of LSIPs along three Yang meridians as well as Ren and Du meridians. *Acupunct. Res.* **18**(2), 98–103.

Liu, J.L. (1989) Observation of rabbit "Neiguan" point area of skin resistance measurement and its influencing factors. *Chin. Acupunct. Moxibustion* **9**(2), 36–38.

Nakatani, Y. (1956) The whole picture of Ryodoraku. *Kampo Clin.* **3**(7), 54.

Shen, J., Kong, E.S., Xu, B., *et al.* (2004) Development of needle sensor for Chinese medicine and related multi-channel measuring instrument. *J. Transducer Tech.* **23**(12), 38.

Yang, H.Y., Xia, J.S., Gu, X.J., *et al.* (1997) The research and application of the dynamic testing system of point skin resistance. *Beijing Biomed. Eng. J. Transducer Tech.* **16**(1), 41.

Wang, Z.J. and Ren, X. (2002) Development of the calcium sensing needle. *J. Transducer Tech.* **21**(3), 31.

Wang, Z.J, Ren, X. and Lu, R. (2003) The study of a temperature sensing needle and an instrument with two channels for measuring temperature. *J. Wuhan Univ. Tech.* **25**(5), 53.

Wei, J.Z., Zhou, Y., Shen, X.Y., *et al.* (2003) Volt-ampere characteristics and functional specificity of acupoints. *Shanghai J. Acupunct. Moxibustion* **22**(9), 18–20.

Zhang, M.Z. (1995) The exploration of methods for electrical measurement of meridian points. *J. Anhui Tradit. Chin. Med. Coll.* **14**(3), 35.

Zheng, Z.L., Zhang, L.J., Yu, W.Y., *et al.* (1958a) The amount of the conductivity of skin acupuncture points and the determination of the normal temperature and its distribution in the whole body. *Shanghai J. Liaoning J. Tradit. Chin. Med.* **12**, 33–37.

Zheng, Z.L., Yu, W.Y., Wu, D.Z., *et al.* (1958b) Electrode area, the skin contact pressure and contact time on the conductivity of the amount of skin acupuncture points. *Shanghai J. Liaoning J. Tradit. Chin. Med.* **12**, 38–41.

Chapter 15

Electrical Acupuncture

Abstract

Electro-Acupuncture therapy is acupuncture based on the standard acupuncture treatment principles of Chinese Medicine. The history of applying Electro-Acupuncture in China was relatively short. Electro-Acupuncture is different from the manual stimulation of acupuncture needling since it is casting its effects to a much wider area. As the development of Electro-Acupuncture equipment continues to progress, basic research has become more serious. There are many types of Electro-Acupuncture equipment, which will be introduced in this chapter.

Keywords: Electro-Acupuncture; Electrical Stimulation.

15.1 Clinical Application of Electrical Acupuncture (EA) and Related Issues

Electro-Acupuncture (EA) therapy is acupuncture based on the standard acupuncture treatment principles of Chinese Medicine.

Chinese Acupuncture treatment was introduced to Europe in the 17th century and attracted the interest of many practicing clinicians. A French doctor, Louis Berlioz, put forward the idea of using electrical current to assist acupuncture in 1810. He thought that basing on the foundation of acupuncture therapy a stimulating current generated by a dry cell could strengthen its treatment effect. Thereafter, a few doctors from Italy, Japan and France continued to carry out EA related clinical research. In June 1915, Dr. Davis of the UK published an article in the *Bristol Journal of Internal and Surgical Medicines* on his treatment experience of EA technique to treat several hundred cases of sciatica and other types of neuritis (Chen and Cai, 1959). Later the most influential figure would be Dr. Reinhold Voll of Germany, who created the Voll EA (Elektroakupunktur nach Dr. Voll, EAV), whose characteristic feature is applied metal plate electrodes on the acupoint to set up a circuit for treatment, using a low frequency pulse. Voll's EA application and relevant research involved therapy as well as diagnosis. He created the acupoint resistance quantitative measurement method and discovered that the diagnostic significance of different measurements, which was also applied to evaluate treatment effects (Li and Zhao, 1994).

The history of applying EA in China was relatively late. According to records, Zhu Longyu of Shanxi was the earliest one who put forward EA treatment method in the 1050s (1953) of the last Century, and developed an EA machine for clinical use. In 1956, he found that EA has significant analgesic effect. As the development of EA equipment was continuously improving, basic research became more serious. The EA equipment could be divided into the following types: "Beep electric acupuncture device, transistor EA instrument, and Pulsed electric acupuncture device. The former two types were seldom used today. The basic equipment of today is the modulated pulse EA instrument, regulated pulse EA instrument, phonic EA, etc.

As a new therapy method, EA is different from the manual stimulation of acupuncture needling. Electrical current itself as a special kind of stimulation could affect the whole human body. Though the result of these observations is confined by historical conditions and objectivity is relatively weak, it still deserves to be used for reference today and merit our attention. Influenced by the use of EA in the West and its application experience (or relevant theory), when China begins to apply EA, it was initially theorized that through electrical current stimulation on the local receptors or peripheral nerve ending, the nerve trunk would transmit the message to the cerebral center where it is based on, producing a kind of modulation effect, overcoming the original uncoordinated phenomenon and achieving the treatment result. However, how important is the acupoint? How do the different points differ from one another on EA? In one study involving 611 patients with different morbidities, standard EA treatment was given and results were compared:

(1) The treatment effects were more or less the same on different stimulated parts. The researchers therefore reasoned that the effective area

of the acupoint could not be confined to the local tiny point, but could instead involve a bigger skin area such that while EA was applied, the stimulation would not be confined to that point and relevant nerve trunk alone.

(2) The treatment effect was not significantly related to the needling depth. While applying EA, the depth of insertion is relatively unimportant. As long as the needle touched on the dermis and subcortex, EA gives expected results.

(3) Application of EA to treat neuropsychiatric disease could be closely related to the whole body response.

(4) EA used to treat local pathology unrelated to internal organs, and results could be closely related to local reflex activities.

(5) For the EA treatment of pathologies of internal organs, the effects are probably transmitted via the segments (Zhang, 1957).

15.2 Factors Affecting Effects of Electrical Acupuncture (EA)

EA produces treatment effects through the interactions of many factors. Considerations should include the following: the original organic state of the patient, the acupuncture point, and the EA stimulation parameters.

(1) The organic state of the patient primarily refers to his/her pathological state. If EA is applied to "PC 6", to those with bradycardia, it could speed up their heart rate (Hou, 1989). However when EA applied to those with tachycardia (Wang, 1994) it could have the opposite effect of slowing down their heart rate; moreover, for hypertension patients, EA on PC 6 could lower the blood pressure (Feng *et al.*, 1994), whereas EA on those with low blood pressure could raise the blood pressure (Wun *et al.*, 2000). Applying EA to "ST 36" may stop diarrhea or reverse constipation (Gong and Ge, 1993).

(2) The treatment effect of EA is related to the acupoint stimulated by virtue of the specific treatment influence designated to the meridian point, which are EA stimulation parameters. Different EA current parameters have different bearing on the treatment effect. Weak stimulation initiates reinforcement, while strong stimulation induces reduction. For example, for the control of pain symptoms, strong EA

stimulation (reduction method) would be indicated, and for those with neuroparalysis, mild stimulation (reinforcement method) would be applied. For those with psychological disturbances, the reduction method is used, while for the depressive state, reinforcement method is used.

15.3 Parameters of Electrical Acupuncture (EA)

The difference between EA and traditional acupuncture is that EA relies on both mechanical stimulation, plus the electrical current stimulation. It is therefore necessary to study the electrical current parameters of EA before it could really reveal the difference between the effect of EA and that of traditional acupuncture and its mechanism of action.

Systematic research on EA analgesia (anesthesia) has been done during the 1950s and the 1960s:

(1) Two hundred and twenty six cases of contraceptive tubal ligation operations patients using acupuncture anesthesia with different combined parameters were studied. The results indicated that under the same conditions of the needling strength and waveform, the effect of high frequency acupuncture anesthesia for making an incision was better than low frequency, and the frequency at 800Hz had the most stable effect. During the needling induction period, the anesthesia effect was better when stimulation intensity was increased once every 5 mins, and the dense wave form was better than continuous wave form (Acupuncture anesthesia Collaborative Group, 1977).

(2) When EA is used for analgesia, high frequency (1000 times/min) is used after a 20–30 min induction time, current intensity is gradually increased up to the patient's endurance limit, and two pairs or more nerves were stimulated with the same EA stimulation; this results in the most satisfactory treatment effect (Acupuncture Anesthesia Research unit, 1978a).

(3) When the EA frequency went above 1000hz, there was a depressive effect on A α, A δ and C waves, and the impact on A δ was most significant. It is suggested that for EA with above 1000 Hz frequency, there is no significant increased analgesic effect, and the depressive effect of EA on small nerve fibers was stronger than on thick ones (Acupuncture Anesthesia Research unit, 1978b).

(4) In a study using domestic rabbits to observe the respective influence of different wavelengths (0.05, 0.1, 0.5, 1.0, 2.5, 5.0, 8.0 ms) on the effect of EA anesthesia, the results suggested that with the suitable wavelength, it could make the two factors, viz. current and tension, reach their mutually supportive effect at the lowest value to produce better anesthetic effect (Acupuncture anesthesia research group, 1978).

(5) Under the stimulation frequency of 100times/min, with a continuous waveform, there was no significant difference with the change of voltages during EA anesthesia (Zhang and Wang, 1979).

15.4 Acupoint Characteristics and Their Relationship with the Design and Effect of Electrical Acupuncture (EA)

Studies indicated that acupuncture points have electrical potentials which are different between different points, and that low resistance is more important. It was also observed that the human body, under different healthy and sick conditions, showed acupoints with varying electrical potentials. Generally speaking, potential changes could reflect the health state of the individual.

References

Chen, D.M. and Cai, X.L. (1959) A preliminary study on the electro-acupuncture therapy. *J. Jiangxi Univ. Tradit. Chin. Med.* **1**, 95–102.

Li, Z. and Zhao, H.M. (1994) About Elektroskupanktur nach Voll. *Foreign Med. Sci.* **16**(2), 55–57.

Zhang, C.H. (1957) Preliminary summary of the research and application of skin electroacupuncture. *J. Xian Jiaotong Univ. (Med. Sci.)* **2**, 4–14.

Hou, J. (1989) Research on the influence of experimental slow heart rate by applying EA to domestic rabbit's "PC 6". *Hangzhou Acad. Educ. J.* **3**, 84–86.

Wang, Q. (1994) Applying current pulse to stimulate PC 6, for the treatment of 35 cases of arrhythmia breaking out, the immediate treatment effect initial conclusion. *Shanghai Biomed. Eng.* **3**, 48–49.

Feng, G., Xing, D. and Sun, Q. (1994) The influence of needling on the blood pressure, SOD, LPO and 5 trace elements of kidney failure and narrow hypertension large mouse. *China East West Med. Integr. Mag.* **14**(12), 739–741.

Wun, S., Cao, Y. and Zhang, J. (2000) Needling PC 6 and SP 4 by EA to treat primary low blood pressure, observation of 100 clinical cases. *Acumoxi Clin. Mag.* **16**(2), 34–35.

Gong, S. and Ge, R. (1993) On the clinical treatment effect of needling ST 36 and its mechanism analysis. *Shanxi Agr. Univ. J.* **13**(3), 274–276.

Acupuncture anesthesia Collaborative Group of Beijing Maternity Hospital, the Institute of Psychology, Chinese Academy of Sciences. (1977) Different electrical stimulation parameters on the clinical effectiveness of acupuncture anesthesia. *Acupunct. Res.* **3**, 109–110.

Acupuncture Anesthesia Research unit of Shanghai First People's Hospital. (1978a) The impact of different stimulation parameters and stimulation mode with electrical nerve stimulation on the effect of EA of the same nerve. *Acupunct. Res.* **2**, 46–51.

Acupuncture anesthesia research group of Second Military Medical University. (1978b) The role of electrical stimulation on the peripheral nerve — more than 1000 cycles/sec frequency electroacupuncture on peripheral nerve. *Acupunct. Res.* **2**, 38–41.

Physiological Unit Ningxia Medical College. (1978) The initial observation of the relationship between the pulse width of electrical stimulation with the effect of acupuncture anesthesia. *Acupunct. Res.* **2**, 51–54.

Zhang, J. and Wang, J.S. (1979) The relationship of electroacupuncture stimulation parameters and the effect of acupuncture anesthesia. *Acupunct. Res.* **1**, 1–7.

Index